Pharmacology for Nursing Students & the NCLEX

A Complete Workbook

Mastering Drug Classes, Mechanisms, and Clinical Applications

for Nursing School and the NCLEX

Dr. David P. Zapencki

DNP, MSN/Ed, CNE, CCRN

Professional Development Publishing

Pharmacology for Nursing Students & the NCLEX

Published by Professional Development Publishing

ISBN 978-1-971135-06-9 (Paperback)

ISBN 978-1-971135-07-6 (eBook)

Table of Contents

Preface

Welcome to Pharmacology for Nursing Students & the NCLEX. This comprehensive resource was designed with one primary goal in mind: to help you master the pharmacological knowledge and clinical reasoning skills essential for safe, effective nursing practice and NCLEX success.

Why This Workbook?

Pharmacology is one of the most challenging and critically important subjects in nursing education. Every day, nurses make medication-related decisions that directly impact patient safety. A single error—wrong dose, wrong route, missed interaction—can have devastating consequences. Yet pharmacology courses often present an overwhelming volume of information: hundreds of drugs, complex mechanisms, and countless nursing considerations.

This workbook takes a different approach. Rather than simply cataloging medications, it focuses on the principles, patterns, and clinical reasoning that will serve you throughout your career. By understanding drug classes, mechanisms of action, and the rationale behind nursing interventions, you'll develop the critical thinking skills needed to manage any medication safely—even ones you've never encountered before.

How This Workbook Is Organized

The ten chapters progress logically from foundational concepts to specialized applications:

- Chapter 1 establishes the pharmacokinetic and pharmacodynamic principles underlying all drug therapy.
- Chapters 2-9 cover major body systems and drug classes, emphasizing the medications most frequently encountered in clinical practice and on the NCLEX.
- Chapter 10 addresses special populations and high-alert medications, integrating concepts from earlier chapters with a focus on safety and error prevention.

Each chapter includes:

- Clear learning objectives to guide your study
- Comprehensive content organized by drug class
- Clinical pearls highlighting key nursing considerations
- BLACK BOX warnings for medications with serious safety concerns

- Memory aids to help you retain critical information
- Twenty NCLEX-style practice questions with detailed rationales

About the Practice Questions

The 200 practice questions in this workbook were carefully crafted to reflect current NCLEX-RN test plan priorities. They emphasize clinical judgment, patient safety, and the application of pharmacological principles to real-world scenarios. The detailed rationales explain not only why the correct answer is right, but also why the incorrect options are wrong—a crucial skill for NCLEX success.

As you work through these questions, resist the urge to simply memorize answers. Instead, focus on understanding the underlying principles. Ask yourself: Why is this the correct nursing action? What could go wrong? What would I monitor? This deeper engagement will serve you far better than rote memorization.

Using This Workbook Effectively

For maximum benefit, I recommend the following approach:

- Read actively. Don't just skim—engage with the material. Highlight key points, take notes, and create your own connections between concepts.
- Study drug classes, not just individual drugs. Understanding the "-olol" suffix tells you about all beta-blockers, not just metoprolol.
- Focus on nursing implications. Knowing a drug's mechanism is important, but knowing what to assess, monitor, and teach is essential.
- Practice application. Complete the practice questions under test-like conditions, then thoroughly review the rationales.
- Connect to clinical experience. When you encounter medications in clinical practice, relate them back to what you've learned.

A Note on Medication Safety

Throughout this workbook, you'll encounter repeated emphasis on safety: the Rights of Medication Administration, high-alert medications, drug interactions, and adverse effects requiring intervention. This emphasis is intentional. Medication errors remain a leading cause of preventable patient harm, and nurses serve as the final checkpoint before a medication reaches a patient.

Never hesitate to question an order that seems incorrect. Never bypass safety systems designed to catch errors. Never assume—always verify. The habits you develop as a student will shape your practice as a nurse.

Acknowledgments

This workbook represents years of clinical experience, teaching, and observation of what helps nursing students succeed. I am grateful to the countless students whose questions and struggles have shaped my understanding of how to teach pharmacology effectively, and to my nursing colleagues whose dedication to patient safety inspires me daily.

Final Thoughts

Pharmacology can seem overwhelming, but it doesn't have to be. With systematic study, clinical reasoning, and a commitment to patient safety, you can master this essential content. This workbook provides the tools—your dedication provides the rest.

I wish you every success in your nursing education and your future career. The patients whose lives you will touch are fortunate to have you as their advocate.

Dr. David P. Zapencki, DNP, MSN/Ed, CNE, CCRN
2026

CHAPTER 1

Foundations of Pharmacology

1.1 Learning Objectives

By the end of this chapter, you will be able to:

- Define key pharmacology terms including pharmacokinetics, pharmacodynamics, and therapeutic index
- Explain the four processes of pharmacokinetics: absorption, distribution, metabolism, and excretion (ADME)
- Describe how pharmacodynamic principles determine drug action and effect
- Identify factors that influence drug response in individual patients
- Recognize common drug interactions and their clinical significance
- Apply medication safety principles to prevent adverse drug events
- Differentiate between generic and brand drug names

1.2 Why Pharmacology Matters

Pharmacology is the study of how drugs interact with living systems. For nurses, pharmacology knowledge is not optional—it is essential for safe practice. Every time you administer a medication, you are making clinical judgments about whether the drug is appropriate, whether the dose is correct, whether the timing is right, and whether the patient is responding as expected.

Medication errors are among the most common and preventable causes of patient harm in healthcare. According to the National Academies of Sciences, Engineering, and Medicine, medication errors harm at least 1.5 million people annually in the United States (National Academies of Sciences, Engineering, and Medicine, 2007). As nurses, we are often the last line of defense before a medication reaches the patient.

The Nurse's Role in Medication Management

Nurses do far more than simply administer medications. The nursing role includes:

Assessment: Evaluating whether a medication is appropriate for this patient at this time. Is the patient allergic? Are there contraindications? Are the vital signs stable enough for this medication?

Administration: Applying the "rights" of medication administration—right patient, right drug, right dose, right route, right time, and right documentation.

Monitoring: Observing for therapeutic effects and adverse effects. Is the medication working? Is the patient experiencing side effects?

Education: Teaching patients about their medications—what they are for, how to take them, what side effects to watch for, and when to seek help.

Advocacy: Speaking up when something does not seem right. Questioning orders that appear incorrect. Communicating concerns to prescribers.

Connecting Pharmacology to Clinical Judgment

Pharmacology knowledge directly supports clinical judgment. When you understand how a drug works, you can:

- Anticipate expected effects and recognize when something is wrong
- Understand why certain monitoring is required
- Explain medications to patients in meaningful ways
- Recognize drug interactions before they cause harm
- Make informed decisions about PRN medication administration

The NCSBN Clinical Judgment Measurement Model applies directly to medication management (National Council of State Boards of Nursing, 2019).

1.3 Essential Pharmacology Terminology

Before diving into pharmacokinetics and pharmacodynamics, you need to understand the language of pharmacology.

Drug Nomenclature

Chemical Name: The precise scientific name describing the drug's molecular structure. Example: N-acetyl-p-aminophenol. You will rarely use chemical names in clinical practice.

Generic Name: The official, nonproprietary name assigned by the United States Adopted Names Council. This is the name you should learn and use. Example: acetaminophen.

Brand Name (Trade Name): The proprietary name given by the manufacturer. Brand names are capitalized. Example: Tylenol®. The same generic drug may have multiple brand names.

Clinical Pearl: Always learn the generic name first. Brand names change; generic names do not.

Key Pharmacology Terms

Pharmacokinetics: What the body does to the drug—how the drug is absorbed, distributed, metabolized, and excreted. Think of it as the drug's journey through the body.

Pharmacodynamics: What the drug does to the body—how the drug produces its effects at the cellular and molecular level.

Onset of Action: The time it takes for a drug to begin producing its effect after administration.

Peak Effect: The time at which the drug reaches its maximum concentration and effect.

Duration of Action: The length of time the drug produces its therapeutic effect.

Half-Life ($t_{1/2}$): The time required for the plasma concentration of a drug to decrease by 50%. Half-life determines dosing frequency.

Steady State: The point at which drug intake equals drug elimination, resulting in a stable plasma concentration. Typically reached after 4-5 half-lives.

Therapeutic Range: The range of drug concentrations in the blood that produces the desired effect without causing toxicity.

Therapeutic Index: The ratio between the toxic dose and the therapeutic dose. A narrow therapeutic index means there is little margin between effective and toxic doses. Examples include digoxin, lithium, warfarin, and aminoglycosides.

Loading Dose: A larger initial dose given to quickly achieve therapeutic levels, followed by smaller maintenance doses.

Maintenance Dose: The regular dose given to maintain therapeutic levels after the loading dose.

1.4 Pharmacokinetics: ADME

Pharmacokinetics describes the movement of drugs through the body. The four key processes are Absorption, Distribution, Metabolism, and Excretion—commonly abbreviated as ADME.

Absorption

Absorption is the movement of a drug from its site of administration into the bloodstream. Several factors affect absorption:

Route of Administration: Different routes have different absorption characteristics.

- Intravenous (IV): Bypasses absorption entirely—100% bioavailability. Used when rapid onset is needed.
- Intramuscular (IM): Absorption depends on blood flow to the muscle. Generally faster than subcutaneous.
- Subcutaneous (SubQ): Slower absorption than IM. Used for drugs needing sustained release like insulin.
- Oral (PO): Most common but most variable. Affected by first-pass effect, food, pH, and GI motility.
- Sublingual/Buccal: Absorbed through oral mucosa, bypassing first-pass metabolism.
- Transdermal: Absorbed through the skin. Provides sustained, controlled release.
- Inhalation: Rapid absorption through large surface area of lungs.

Bioavailability: The percentage of administered drug that reaches systemic circulation in active form. IV drugs have 100% bioavailability.

First-Pass Effect: When drugs are absorbed from the GI tract, they first travel to the liver via the portal circulation. The liver may metabolize a significant portion before it reaches systemic circulation.

Distribution

Distribution is the movement of drug from the bloodstream to body tissues.

Blood Flow: Highly perfused organs (heart, liver, kidneys, brain) receive drugs quickly.

Protein Binding: Many drugs bind to plasma proteins, primarily albumin. Only the unbound (free) drug is pharmacologically active.

Clinical Pearl: Patients with low albumin (malnutrition, liver disease) may have higher free drug levels and increased toxicity risk.

Blood-Brain Barrier: A selective barrier that protects the brain. Only lipid-soluble, non-ionized, unbound drugs cross easily.

Placental Barrier: Most drugs can cross the placenta—critical when caring for pregnant patients.

Metabolism (Biotransformation)

Metabolism is the chemical alteration of drugs by the body, primarily in the liver.

CYP450 Enzymes: A family of liver enzymes that metabolize many drugs. CYP3A4 metabolizes about 50% of all drugs.

- Enzyme Inducers: Increase CYP450 activity, causing faster metabolism. Examples: phenytoin, carbamazepine, rifampin, St. John's wort.
- Enzyme Inhibitors: Decrease CYP450 activity, causing slower metabolism. Examples: ketoconazole, erythromycin, grapefruit juice, cimetidine.

Prodrugs: Inactive compounds that must be metabolized to their active form. Example: codeine is converted to morphine by CYP2D6.

First-Order vs. Zero-Order Kinetics:

- First-Order: Constant percentage metabolized per unit time. Most drugs follow this.
- Zero-Order: Constant amount metabolized regardless of concentration. Alcohol follows this—small dose increases cause large level increases.

Excretion

Excretion is the removal of drugs and metabolites from the body. The kidneys are the primary route.

Renal Excretion: Most drugs and metabolites are excreted by the kidneys through glomerular filtration and tubular secretion.

Clinical Pearl: Patients with renal impairment may require dose adjustments. Always check creatinine clearance or GFR for renally excreted drugs.

Hepatic Excretion: Some drugs are excreted in bile. Some undergo enterohepatic recirculation, prolonging their duration.

Other Routes: Minor routes include lungs (volatile anesthetics), sweat, saliva, and breast milk.

1.5 Pharmacodynamics: How Drugs Work

Pharmacodynamics describes what the drug does to the body.

Receptor Theory

Most drugs produce effects by interacting with receptors—specific protein molecules on or in cells.

Agonists: Bind to receptors and activate them, producing a response. Example: Albuterol is a beta-2 agonist causing bronchodilation.

Antagonists: Bind to receptors but do not activate them—they block. Example: Propranolol is a beta blocker.

Partial Agonists: Produce partial response. Example: Buprenorphine is a partial opioid agonist.

Affinity: How strongly a drug binds to its receptor.

Efficacy: The ability of a drug to produce a response once bound to a receptor.

Potency: The amount of drug required to produce a given effect. A more potent drug works at lower doses.

Therapeutic Index

Therapeutic Index (TI): The ratio of toxic dose to therapeutic dose. TI = TD50/ED50

- Wide TI: Large margin of safety. Example: penicillin.
- Narrow TI: Small margin between therapeutic and toxic. Requires careful monitoring. Examples: digoxin, lithium, warfarin, phenytoin, theophylline, aminoglycosides.

Factors Affecting Drug Response

Age: Neonates have immature hepatic/renal function. Older adults have decreased function.

Body Weight: Larger patients may need higher doses.

Genetics (Pharmacogenomics): Genetic variations affect metabolism. Some patients are "rapid" or "poor" metabolizers.

Disease States: Liver disease impairs metabolism. Kidney disease impairs excretion.

Tolerance: Decreased response after repeated exposure, requiring higher doses.

1.6 Drug Interactions

Drug interactions occur when one drug affects the action of another.

Types of Interactions

Pharmacokinetic Interactions: One drug affects ADME of another.

- Absorption: Antacids can decrease absorption of many drugs.
- Metabolism: CYP450 inducers or inhibitors change metabolism of other drugs.

Pharmacodynamic Interactions: Drugs with similar or opposing mechanisms interact at the receptor level.

- Additive: Combined effect equals sum of individual effects.
- Synergistic: Combined effect greater than sum.
- Antagonistic: One drug reduces effect of another.

High-Risk Interactions

Warfarin: Numerous interactions. Many drugs increase bleeding risk; others decrease anticoagulation. Close INR monitoring essential.

Serotonin Syndrome: Combining serotonergic drugs can be life-threatening. Avoid MAOIs with SSRIs.

QT Prolongation: Many drugs prolong QT interval. Combining them increases risk of fatal arrhythmias.

CNS Depression: Combining CNS depressants (opioids, benzodiazepines, alcohol) can cause respiratory depression and death.

Drug-Food Interactions

Grapefruit Juice: Inhibits CYP3A4, increasing blood levels of statins, CCBs, and others.

Vitamin K Foods: Affect warfarin. Maintain consistent intake.

Tyramine Foods: Can cause hypertensive crisis with MAOIs. Avoid aged cheeses, cured meats.

Clinical Pearl: Always ask patients about herbal supplements and OTC medications.

1.7 Adverse Drug Reactions

Adverse drug reactions (ADRs) are harmful, unintended effects of medications.

Types of Adverse Reactions

Side Effects: Predictable, dose-related effects. Example: drowsiness with antihistamines.

Toxic Effects: Harmful effects when drug levels exceed therapeutic range.

Allergic Reactions: Immune-mediated. Range from rash to anaphylaxis.

- Type I (Immediate): IgE-mediated. Urticaria, angioedema, anaphylaxis. Onset within minutes.
- Type IV (Delayed): T-cell mediated. Contact dermatitis. Onset 48-72 hours.

Idiosyncratic Reactions: Unusual, unpredictable responses. Often genetically determined.

Drug-Induced Organ Toxicity

- Hepatotoxicity: Acetaminophen overdose, isoniazid, statins
- Nephrotoxicity: NSAIDs, aminoglycosides, vancomycin, contrast dye
- Ototoxicity: Aminoglycosides, loop diuretics, cisplatin

Black Box Warnings

The FDA's most serious warning. Examples:

- Fluoroquinolones: Tendon rupture, peripheral neuropathy
- Antidepressants: Increased suicidal thinking in young adults
- Opioids: Respiratory depression, especially with benzodiazepines

1.8 Medication Safety Principles

The Rights of Medication Administration

Right Patient: Use two patient identifiers.

Right Drug: Verify medication matches order. Check for look-alike, sound-alike drugs.

Right Dose: Verify dose is appropriate. Question unusually high or low doses.

Right Route: Confirm ordered route. Never crush extended-release medications.

Right Time: Administer within acceptable time window.

Right Documentation: Document promptly and accurately.

Right Reason: Understand why patient is receiving this medication.

Right Response: Monitor for therapeutic and adverse effects.

High-Alert Medications

High-alert medications carry increased risk of harm when used in error (ISMP, 2024):

- Anticoagulants (heparin, warfarin, DOACs)
- Opioids
- Insulin
- Sedatives/anesthetics
- Neuromuscular blocking agents
- Chemotherapy drugs
- Concentrated electrolytes (potassium chloride, hypertonic saline)

Look-Alike, Sound-Alike (LASA) Drugs

- Hydroxyzine vs. hydralazine
- Celebrex vs. Celexa vs. Cerebyx
- Metformin vs. metronidazole

Prevention: Use tall-man lettering (hydrOXYzine vs. hydrALAZINE), verify with indication.

1.9 Special Considerations

Pediatric Patients

Children are not small adults. Considerations:

- Immature hepatic enzymes and renal function
- Different body composition (higher water content)
- Weight-based dosing (mg/kg) is standard

Geriatric Patients

Older adults have physiological changes affecting drug response:

- Decreased gastric acid and motility (altered absorption)
- Decreased lean body mass, increased fat (altered distribution)
- Decreased hepatic and renal function
- Increased sensitivity to medications, especially CNS effects

Beers Criteria: List of potentially inappropriate medications for older adults (AGS, 2023).

Clinical Pearl: Start low, go slow.

Pregnancy and Lactation

The Pregnancy and Lactation Labeling Rule (PLLR) require narrative descriptions of risks (FDA, 2014).

Known teratogens: Isotretinoin, warfarin, valproic acid, methotrexate, ACE inhibitors.

Hepatic and Renal Impairment

Patients with liver disease: decreased metabolism, decreased protein binding.

Patients with kidney disease: decreased excretion, drug accumulation, increased toxicity risk.

1.10 Applying Pharmacology Knowledge

Before administering any medication, assess: allergies, current medications, relevant labs, vital signs, contraindications.

Patient education should include: drug name, purpose, how to take it, side effects, warning signs, interactions to avoid.

1.11 Chapter Summary

Pharmacology provides the foundation for safe medication administration. Key concepts:

- Pharmacokinetics (ADME): How the body handles drugs
- Pharmacodynamics: How drugs produce effects through receptors
- Therapeutic Index: Margin between therapeutic and toxic doses
- Drug Interactions: Can enhance or reduce drug effects
- Medication Safety: Apply the rights; know high-alert and LASA drugs
- Special Populations: Adjust for age, pregnancy, organ impairment

1.12 Practice Questions

Directions: Select the best answer for each question. Answers and rationales are in the Answer Key.

1. A nurse is reviewing a medication order for a patient with liver cirrhosis. Which pharmacokinetic process is most likely to be significantly impaired?

A. Absorption from the GI tract

B. Distribution to adipose tissue

C. Hepatic metabolism of medications

D. Renal excretion of metabolites

2. A patient is receiving warfarin and is started on rifampin. The nurse should anticipate that rifampin will:

A. Increase the anticoagulant effect of warfarin

B. Decrease the anticoagulant effect of warfarin

C. Have no effect on warfarin therapy

D. Cause an allergic reaction when combined

3. Digoxin has a narrow therapeutic index. This means:

A. The drug is safe to give at any dose

B. There is a large margin between therapeutic and toxic dose

C. There is a small margin between therapeutic and toxic dose

D. The drug must be given intravenously

4. Which statement indicates the patient understands half-life?

A. The medication will be completely gone in one half-life

B. After one half-life, half will be eliminated from my body

C. Half-life tells me how long until it starts working

D. I should take half the dose if I have side effects

5. A patient asks why levothyroxine must be taken on an empty stomach. This addresses which process?

A. Absorption

B. Distribution

C. Metabolism

D. Excretion

6. A patient takes both warfarin and aspirin. This is an example of which interaction?

A. Antagonistic interaction

B. Additive interaction

C. Synergistic interaction

D. Idiosyncratic interaction

7. An older adult develops new confusion after starting a medication. The nurse should first:

A. Assume the confusion is related to aging

B. Consider it may be an adverse drug reaction

C. Administer a PRN sedative

D. Wait to see if it resolves

8. A patient on phenytoin starts a CYP450 inhibitor. The nurse should monitor for:

A. Decreased phenytoin levels and seizures

B. Increased phenytoin levels and toxicity

C. No change in phenytoin levels

D. Allergic reaction to phenytoin

9. Which patient is at highest risk for adverse drug reactions?

A. 25-year-old on one medication

B. 45-year-old on metformin only

C. 78-year-old on eight medications

D. 30-year-old pregnant on prenatal vitamins

10. Which statement about IV administration is correct?

A. IV meds have approximately 50% bioavailability

B. IV meds bypass the first-pass effect completely

C. IV meds must be metabolized before becoming active

D. IV meds are always safer than oral

11. Aminoglycosides require peak/trough monitoring because they:

A. Have a wide therapeutic index

B. Have a narrow therapeutic index

C. Are not absorbed when given orally

D. Require hepatic activation

12. Grapefruit juice increases blood levels of certain medications by:

A. Increasing renal excretion

B. Inhibiting intestinal CYP3A4 enzymes

C. Increasing gastric acid production

D. Enhancing protein binding

13. A patient on St. John's Wort should be most concerned if also taking:

A. Acetaminophen

B. Oral contraceptives

C. Calcium supplements

D. Multivitamins

14. Hives and difficulty breathing after penicillin is best described as:

A. A predictable side effect

B. An idiosyncratic reaction

C. A Type I hypersensitivity reaction

D. A Type IV hypersensitivity reaction

15. Pediatric medication doses should be calculated based on:

A. Adult dose divided by child's age

B. Child's weight in kilograms

C. Adult dose if child weighs over 50 pounds

D. Child's height

16. In CKD stage 4, the nurse should be most concerned about accumulation of:

A. Drugs metabolized primarily by the liver

B. Drugs that are highly protein-bound

C. Drugs excreted primarily by the kidneys

D. Drugs with large volumes of distribution

17. A patient on opioids and benzodiazepines should be monitored for:

A. Serotonin syndrome

B. Respiratory depression

C. QT prolongation

D. Hypertensive crisis

18. Which statement shows understanding of steady state?

A. Steady state is reached after the first dose

B. Steady state occurs when intake equals elimination

C. Steady state means the drug reached toxic levels

D. Steady state is only important for IV medications

19. Extended-release formulations:

A. Work faster than immediate-release versions

B. Provide more consistent blood levels with less frequent dosing

C. Are always more effective than immediate-release versions

D. Can be crushed for patients with difficulty swallowing

20. The most important action in medication reconciliation is to:

A. Document only prescription medications

B. Include over-the-counter medications and supplements

C. Rely on patient's memory for names and doses

D. Skip medications from other providers

CHAPTER 2

Cardiovascular Medications

2.1 Learning Objectives

By the end of this chapter, you will be able to:

- Identify the major classes of cardiovascular medications and their mechanisms of action
- Explain the therapeutic uses and nursing considerations for antihypertensive medications
- Describe the differences between anticoagulants and antiplatelet agents
- Recognize the signs and symptoms of digoxin toxicity
- Apply appropriate monitoring parameters for patients receiving cardiovascular medications
- Differentiate between the classes of antiarrhythmic drugs
- Educate patients about lipid-lowering therapy and lifestyle modifications

2.2 Overview of Cardiovascular Pharmacology

Cardiovascular diseases remain the leading cause of death worldwide. Nurses play a critical role in administering cardiovascular medications safely, monitoring for effects, and educating patients. This chapter covers antihypertensives, antianginal agents, antiarrhythmics, cardiac glycosides, anticoagulants, antiplatelets, and lipid-lowering agents.

2.3 Antihypertensive Medications

Hypertension affects nearly half of American adults. Goal: <130/80 mmHg for most adults.

ACE Inhibitors

Mechanism: Block conversion of angiotensin I to angiotensin II, causing vasodilation and decreased aldosterone.

Drugs: Lisinopril, enalapril, captopril, ramipril. *Memory Tip:* End in "-pril"

Uses: Hypertension, heart failure, post-MI, diabetic nephropathy (renal protection).

Nursing Considerations: Monitor BP, potassium (hyperkalemia risk), renal function. First-dose hypotension possible—start low.

Adverse Effects: Dry persistent cough (bradykinin accumulation—most common reason for discontinuation), hyperkalemia, angioedema (rare but life-threatening).

Contraindications: Pregnancy (teratogenic), history of angioedema, bilateral renal artery stenosis.

Clinical Pearl: If patient develops dry cough on ACE inhibitor, provider may switch to ARB.

Angiotensin II Receptor Blockers (ARBs)

Drugs: Losartan, valsartan, irbesartan, olmesartan. *Memory Tip:* End in "-sartan"

Similar effects to ACE inhibitors but do not cause cough (no bradykinin effect). Do not combine with ACE inhibitors.

Beta-Adrenergic Blockers

Mechanism: Block beta receptors, decreasing heart rate, contractility, and BP.

Cardioselective (Beta-1): Metoprolol, atenolol, bisoprolol—preferred in COPD/diabetes

Nonselective: Propranolol, carvedilol, labetalol

Memory Tip: End in "-olol"

Uses: Hypertension, heart failure (specific agents), angina, arrhythmias, post-MI, migraine prophylaxis.

Nursing Considerations: Check HR before giving—hold if < 60 bpm. Check BP—hold if SBP < 90 mmHg. NEVER discontinue abruptly (rebound hypertension, angina, MI). Taper over 1-2 weeks.

Adverse Effects: Bradycardia, hypotension, fatigue, bronchospasm (avoid nonselective in asthma), masks hypoglycemia symptoms in diabetics.

Clinical Pearl: Cardioselective agents preferred in patients with mild COPD or diabetes.

Calcium Channel Blockers

Dihydropyridines (primarily vasodilation): Amlodipine, nifedipine. *Memory Tip:* End in "-dipine"

Non-dihydropyridines (vasodilation + cardiac effects): Diltiazem, verapamil

Nursing: Monitor BP/HR. Diltiazem/verapamil—check HR, hold if < 60. Avoid grapefruit juice. Do NOT combine verapamil/diltiazem with beta blockers (severe bradycardia risk).

Adverse Effects: Dihydropyridines—peripheral edema (ankles), headache, flushing. Non-dihydropyridines—bradycardia, constipation (verapamil).

Diuretics

Thiazides (HCTZ, chlorthalidone): First line for HTN. Cause hypokalemia, hyperglycemia, hyperuricemia (gout), hypercalcemia.

Loop Diuretics (Furosemide, bumetanide): Most potent. Cause hypokalemia, hypomagnesemia, hypocalcemia, ototoxicity with rapid IV push.

Clinical Pearl: "Thiazides keep calcium" (hyperCa), loops lose it (hypoCa). Furosemide IV works in 5 min; oral takes 30-60 min.

Potassium-Sparing (Spironolactone, eplerenone, triamterene): Cause HYPERKALEMIA. Avoid K+ supplements and salt substitutes. Spironolactone causes gynecomastia.

2.4 Antianginal Medications: Nitrates

Mechanism: Convert to nitric oxide → vasodilation → decreased preload → decreased cardiac workload.

Drugs: Nitroglycerin (sublingual, patch, IV), isosorbide mononitrate, isosorbide dinitrate.

Sublingual Nitroglycerin Instructions

- Sit or lie down before taking (prevents falls from hypotension)
- Place tablet under tongue—do not swallow
- May repeat every 5 minutes × 3 doses
- Call 911 if pain persists after 3 doses—may be MI
- Store in original dark glass container; replace every 6 months
- Should cause slight burning/tingling—if not, may be expired

Nitroglycerin Patches

- Apply to clean, dry, hairless skin; rotate sites
- Remove for 10-12 hours daily (usually at night) to prevent tolerance
- Remove before MRI or defibrillation

Adverse Effects: Headache (very common), hypotension, dizziness, flushing.

CRITICAL CONTRAINDICATION: NEVER give with phosphodiesterase-5 inhibitors (sildenafil/Viagra, tadalafil/Cialis)—causes severe, life-threatening hypotension!

Clinical Pearl: Always ask about erectile dysfunction medications before giving nitrates.

2.5 Antiarrhythmic Medications

Class I (Sodium Channel Blockers): Quinidine, lidocaine, flecainide

Class II (Beta Blockers): Metoprolol, esmolol

Class III (Potassium Channel Blockers): Amiodarone, sotalol, dofetilide

Class IV (Calcium Channel Blockers): Diltiazem, verapamil

Amiodarone

Most commonly used antiarrhythmic. Effective for atrial and ventricular arrhythmias. Very long half-life (40-55 days).

Serious Adverse Effects (requires monitoring):

- Pulmonary toxicity (fibrosis)—monitor chest X-ray, pulmonary function
- Hepatotoxicity—monitor LFTs
- Thyroid dysfunction (hypo- or hyperthyroidism)—monitor thyroid function
- Corneal deposits, photosensitivity, blue-gray skin discoloration
- QT prolongation

Clinical Pearl: Amiodarone is called a "dirty drug" because of many effects, but highly effective when others fail.

Adenosine

First-line for SVT. Given as rapid IV push followed by flush. Very short half-life (< 10 seconds).

Warn patient: may feel chest discomfort or "impending doom" (causes transient asystole).

2.6 Cardiac Glycosides: Digoxin

Mechanism: Positive inotrope (↑ contraction strength), negative chronotrope (↓ HR), negative dromotrope (↓ AV conduction).

Uses: Heart failure (improves symptoms, not survival), atrial fibrillation (rate control).

Therapeutic Range: 0.5-2.0 ng/mL (narrow therapeutic index).

Nursing Considerations

- Check APICAL pulse for ONE FULL MINUTE before giving
- Hold if pulse < 60 bpm in adults (< 70 children, < 90-110 infants)
- Check potassium level—hypokalemia increases toxicity risk
- Monitor digoxin levels (draw 6-8 hours after dose), renal function

Digoxin Toxicity

Risk Factors: Hypokalemia (most common), hypomagnesemia, hypercalcemia, renal impairment, drug interactions.

Signs/Symptoms:

- GI: Anorexia (often FIRST sign), nausea, vomiting
- Visual: Blurred vision, yellow-green halos around lights (xanthopsia)
- Cardiac: Bradycardia, heart block, arrhythmias

- Neurological: Fatigue, weakness, confusion

Treatment: Stop digoxin, correct electrolytes (especially K+), cardiac monitoring. Severe toxicity: Digoxin immune fab (Digibind).

Drug Interactions: Amiodarone, verapamil, quinidine increase digoxin levels—reduce digoxin dose by 50%.

Clinical Pearl: "Dig toxicity loves low potassium." Always check K+ when patient has new symptoms.

2.7 Anticoagulant Medications

Heparin (Unfractionated)

Mechanism: Enhances antithrombin III activity.

Administration: IV (continuous) or subcutaneous. Cannot give orally.

Monitoring: aPTT (goal 1.5-2.5 × control), platelet count (for HIT).

Adverse Effects: Bleeding, heparin-induced thrombocytopenia (HIT)—low platelets AND paradoxical clotting.

Antidote: Protamine sulfate.

Low Molecular Weight Heparins (LMWH)

Drugs: Enoxaparin (Lovenox), dalteparin.

Advantages: Predictable response, SubQ administration (home use), less monitoring needed, lower HIT risk.

Administration: Deep SubQ in abdomen. Do NOT expel air bubble. Do NOT rub injection site. Rotate sites.

Warfarin (Coumadin)

Mechanism: Inhibits vitamin K-dependent clotting factors (II, VII, IX, X). Takes 3-5 days for full effect.

Monitoring: PT/INR. Goal: 2.0-3.0 (most indications); 2.5-3.5 (mechanical heart valves).

Key Points: Bridge with heparin until INR therapeutic. Many drug/food interactions. Maintain CONSISTENT vitamin K intake (don't avoid, be consistent). Teratogenic—avoid in pregnancy.

Drug Interactions: Increase effect—amiodarone, antibiotics, NSAIDs. Decrease effect—rifampin, vitamin K, St. John's Wort.

Antidote: Vitamin K (phytonadione); severe bleeding—FFP or prothrombin complex concentrate.

Direct Oral Anticoagulants (DOACs)

Drugs: Dabigatran (Pradaxa)—thrombin inhibitor; Rivaroxaban (Xarelto), apixaban (Eliquis), edoxaban—factor Xa inhibitors.

Advantages: Fixed dosing, no routine monitoring, fewer interactions, rapid onset (no bridging needed).

Nursing: Do NOT crush. Rivaroxaban with food. Assess renal function.

Antidotes: Dabigatran—idarucizumab (Praxbind); Factor Xa inhibitors—andexanet alfa.

2.8 Antiplatelet Medications

Aspirin

Mechanism: Irreversibly inhibits COX, blocking platelet aggregation for 7-10 days (life of platelet).

Uses: Acute MI (chew 162-325 mg immediately), secondary prevention (81 mg daily).

P2Y12 Inhibitors

Drugs: Clopidogrel (Plavix), prasugrel, ticagrelor.

Uses: ACS, post-PCI with stent (dual antiplatelet therapy with aspirin).

Notes: Clopidogrel is prodrug—avoid PPIs (reduce effectiveness). Hold 5-7 days before surgery.

Clinical Pearl: Dual antiplatelet therapy (aspirin + P2Y12 inhibitor) is standard after coronary stent placement.

2.9 Lipid-Lowering Medications

Statins (HMG-CoA Reductase Inhibitors)

Drugs: Atorvastatin, rosuvastatin (high intensity); simvastatin, pravastatin (moderate). *Memory Tip:* End in "-statin"

Mechanism: Inhibit cholesterol synthesis. Lower LDL, raise HDL slightly, lower triglycerides.

Administration: Evening preferred for short-acting statins. Avoid grapefruit with simvastatin, lovastatin, atorvastatin.

Monitoring: LFTs (baseline), muscle symptoms.

Adverse Effects: Myopathy (muscle pain/weakness)—can progress to RHABDOMYOLYSIS (muscle breakdown → acute kidney injury). Elevated LFTs, increased glucose.

Rhabdomyolysis Risk Increased With: High doses, drug interactions (gemfibrozil), hypothyroidism, renal impairment.

Clinical Pearl: Teach patients to report unexplained muscle pain, weakness, or dark urine IMMEDIATELY.

Other Lipid-Lowering Agents

Ezetimibe: Inhibits cholesterol absorption. Used with statins.

Bile Acid Sequestrants: Cholestyramine, colesevelam. Give other meds 1 hour before or 4-6 hours after.

Fibrates: Gemfibrozil, fenofibrate. Lower triglycerides. Increase myopathy risk with statins.

PCSK9 Inhibitors: Alirocumab, evolocumab. Injectable; very effective for LDL.

2.10 Heart Failure Medications

First-Line for HFrEF: ACE inhibitors/ARBs, beta blockers (metoprolol succinate, carvedilol, bisoprolol), aldosterone antagonists (spironolactone, eplerenone), loop diuretics.

Sacubitril/Valsartan (Entresto): Superior to ACE inhibitors for survival. Cannot use WITH ACE inhibitors (wait 36 hours).

SGLT2 Inhibitors: Dapagliflozin, empagliflozin. Originally diabetes drugs; improve heart failure outcomes.

2.11 Chapter Summary

Key points for cardiovascular medications:

- Beta blockers: Always check HR; hold if < 60; never stop abruptly
- ACE inhibitors: Monitor for cough, hyperkalemia, angioedema; contraindicated in pregnancy
- Digoxin: Check apical pulse × 1 min; check potassium; know toxicity signs (anorexia, yellow-green halos)
- Anticoagulants: Heparin—aPTT; Warfarin—INR; DOACs—no routine monitoring
- Nitrates: NEVER give with PDE5 inhibitors (sildenafil, tadalafil)
- Statins: Report muscle pain immediately (rhabdomyolysis risk)

2.12 Practice Questions

Directions: Select the best answer for each question.

1. A patient taking lisinopril reports a persistent dry cough. The nurse understands this is caused by:

A. Decreased cardiac output

B. Accumulation of bradykinin

C. Allergic reaction to the medication

D. Development of heart failure

2. Before administering metoprolol, the nurse should check the patient's:

A. Blood glucose level

B. Apical heart rate

C. Potassium level

D. INR

3. A patient on digoxin has a potassium level of 3.0 mEq/L. The nurse should:

A. Administer the digoxin as ordered

B. Hold the digoxin and notify the provider

C. Give extra potassium supplements without an order

D. Recheck the potassium level in 24 hours

4. A nurse caring for a patient receiving IV heparin should monitor which lab value?

A. PT/INR

B. aPTT

C. Platelet count only

D. Hemoglobin

5. A patient taking warfarin asks about diet. The nurse should instruct:

A. Avoid all foods containing vitamin K

B. Maintain consistent intake of vitamin K foods

C. Increase vitamin K intake to counteract medication

D. Take vitamin K supplements daily

6. Which statement indicates the patient needs more teaching about sublingual nitroglycerin?

A. I should sit down before taking this medication

B. I can take up to three tablets, five minutes apart

C. I should call 911 if pain continues after three tablets

D. I can take this with my sildenafil if pain is severe

7. When administering furosemide 40 mg IV push, the most important action is:

A. Administer over at least 1-2 minutes

B. Check blood glucose before administration

C. Verify the patient has eaten breakfast

D. Administer with orange juice

8. A patient receiving amiodarone should be monitored for:

A. Pulmonary toxicity

B. Hypoglycemia

C. Hair loss

D. Weight loss

9. The most important instruction for a patient taking clopidogrel is:

A. Take this medication with antacids

B. You may stop if you feel better

C. Tell all healthcare providers you take this medication

D. This medication should be taken at bedtime only

10. A patient on atorvastatin reports new muscle pain and weakness. The nurse should:

A. Reassure that this is a common harmless side effect

B. Advise increased fluid intake

C. Notify the provider immediately

D. Recommend taking in the morning instead

11. A patient's INR is 4.5 while taking warfarin. The nurse should anticipate:

A. Increasing the warfarin dose

B. Holding warfarin and monitoring for bleeding

C. Administering protamine sulfate

D. Continuing current warfarin dose

12. An early sign of digoxin toxicity is:

A. Hypertension

B. Anorexia

C. Increased appetite

D. Tachycardia

13. A patient is prescribed furosemide and digoxin. The nurse should monitor for:

A. Hyperkalemia

B. Hypokalemia

C. Hypernatremia

D. Hypercalcemia

14. When administering enoxaparin subcutaneously, the nurse should:

A. Aspirate before injecting

B. Massage the site after injection

C. Inject into the abdomen, rotating sites

D. Remove the air bubble before injection

15. A patient on apixaban demonstrates understanding by stating:

A. I need weekly blood tests

B. I should avoid all green leafy vegetables

C. I should not crush this medication

D. I will take vitamin K if I have any bleeding

16. For a patient taking amlodipine, the nurse should report:

A. Heart rate of 72 bpm

B. Blood pressure of 118/76 mmHg

C. New onset of ankle swelling

D. Occasional mild headaches

17. A patient asks why the nitroglycerin patch is removed at night. The nurse explains:

A. To reduce nighttime hypotension

B. To prevent development of tolerance

C. To allow the skin to rest from adhesive

D. To decrease headaches during sleep

18. Which patient should the nurse question before giving a beta blocker?

A. Patient with hypertension and diabetes

B. Patient with heart failure and HR of 68 bpm

C. Patient with asthma and wheezing

D. Patient with angina and BP of 140/88 mmHg

19. A patient receiving tPA for stroke should be monitored most closely for:

A. Hypokalemia

B. Bleeding

C. Bronchospasm

D. Hyperglycemia

20. A patient taking spironolactone should avoid:

A. Calcium supplements

B. Potassium-rich foods and salt substitutes

C. Dairy products

D. Vitamin C supplements

CHAPTER 3

Respiratory Medications

3.1 Learning Objectives

By the end of this chapter, you will be able to:

- Differentiate between short-acting and long-acting bronchodilators
- Explain the mechanisms and nursing considerations for inhaled corticosteroids
- Identify appropriate rescue versus maintenance medications for asthma and COPD
- Describe proper inhaler and nebulizer administration techniques
- Recognize adverse effects of respiratory medications requiring intervention
- Apply the stepwise approach to asthma management
- Educate patients about preventing oral candidiasis with inhaled corticosteroids

3.2 Overview of Respiratory Pharmacology

Respiratory diseases including asthma and COPD affect millions of people. Medications target bronchoconstriction, inflammation, and mucus production. Understanding the difference between rescue (quick-relief) and maintenance (controller) medications is essential for safe nursing practice.

3.3 Bronchodilators

Bronchodilators relax bronchial smooth muscle to open airways. Three main classes: beta-2 agonists, anticholinergics, and methylxanthines.

Short-Acting Beta-2 Agonists (SABAs)

Drugs: Albuterol (Ventolin, ProAir, Proventil), levalbuterol (Xopenex)

Mechanism: Stimulate beta-2 receptors in bronchial smooth muscle → bronchodilation

Uses: RESCUE medication for acute bronchospasm in asthma and COPD. Quick relief of symptoms.

Onset: 5-15 minutes. Duration: 4-6 hours.

Nursing Considerations:

- Teach proper inhaler technique—shake well, exhale fully, inhale slowly while pressing canister

- Wait 1 minute between puffs if multiple puffs ordered
- Rinse mouth after use to reduce local irritation
- If using with inhaled corticosteroid, use SABA first to open airways

Adverse Effects: Tachycardia, palpitations, tremor, nervousness, hypokalemia (with high doses)

Clinical Pearl: If patient needs SABA more than 2 times per week (excluding exercise pre-treatment), asthma is not well controlled—reassess therapy.

Long-Acting Beta-2 Agonists (LABAs)

Drugs: Salmeterol (Serevent), formoterol (Foradil), vilanterol (in Breo)

Mechanism: Same as SABAs but longer duration (12-24 hours)

Uses: MAINTENANCE therapy for asthma and COPD. NOT for acute symptoms.

BLACK BOX WARNING: LABAs increase risk of asthma-related death when used alone. Must ALWAYS be used with inhaled corticosteroid in asthma patients.

Nursing Considerations:

- Never use as rescue medication—onset too slow for acute symptoms
- Always combine with inhaled corticosteroid for asthma
- Available in combination inhalers (e.g., Advair = fluticasone + salmeterol)

Clinical Pearl: Teach patients: "LABAs are for long-term control, SABAs are for short-term rescue."

Anticholinergics (Muscarinic Antagonists)

Short-Acting: Ipratropium (Atrovent)—onset 15-30 min, duration 4-6 hours

Long-Acting: Tiotropium (Spiriva), umeclidinium (Incruse)—duration 24 hours

Mechanism: Block acetylcholine at muscarinic receptors → bronchodilation and decreased secretions

Uses: COPD (first-line), asthma (adjunct). Ipratropium often combined with albuterol (DuoNeb, Combivent).

Adverse Effects: Dry mouth (most common), urinary retention, constipation, blurred vision. Use caution in glaucoma and BPH.

Nursing Considerations:

- Tiotropium (Spiriva): Use HandiHaler device—do not swallow capsules
- Protect eyes from spray (can precipitate acute glaucoma)
- Good oral hygiene and sips of water for dry mouth

Clinical Pearl: In COPD, anticholinergics are often preferred over beta-2 agonists as first-line maintenance.

Methylxanthines

Drug: Theophylline (Theo-24, Elixophyllin)

Mechanism: Phosphodiesterase inhibitor → bronchodilation, mild anti-inflammatory

Uses: Third-line for asthma/COPD when other treatments inadequate. Rarely used due to toxicity.

NARROW THERAPEUTIC INDEX: Therapeutic range 5-15 mcg/mL. Toxicity common.

Adverse Effects: Nausea, vomiting, headache, insomnia, tachycardia. Severe toxicity: seizures, arrhythmias.

Drug Interactions: Many! Cimetidine, fluoroquinolones, macrolides increase levels. Smoking, phenytoin, rifampin decrease levels.

Nursing Considerations:

- Monitor serum theophylline levels
- Take with food to decrease GI upset
- Avoid caffeine (same drug class)
- Report signs of toxicity: persistent vomiting, tremors, rapid heart rate

Clinical Pearl: If patient who smokes on theophylline quits smoking, theophylline levels will INCREASE—may need dose reduction.

3.4 Anti-Inflammatory Agents

Inhaled Corticosteroids (ICS)

Drugs: Fluticasone (Flovent), budesonide (Pulmicort), beclomethasone (QVAR), mometasone (Asmanex)

Mechanism: Decrease airway inflammation, reduce mucus production, decrease bronchial hyperreactivity

Uses: FIRST-LINE MAINTENANCE therapy for persistent asthma. Also used in COPD with frequent exacerbations.

Onset: Days to weeks for full effect. NOT for acute symptoms.

Adverse Effects:

- Oral candidiasis (thrush)—most common local effect
- Dysphonia (hoarseness)
- With high doses/long-term: adrenal suppression, osteoporosis, growth suppression in children, cataracts

Nursing Considerations:

- RINSE MOUTH and spit after each use to prevent thrush
- Use spacer device with MDI to improve delivery and reduce oral deposition

- If using SABA and ICS, use SABA first, wait 5 minutes, then use ICS
- Teach that this is daily maintenance—not rescue

Clinical Pearl: Ask patients to show you their mouth—white patches indicate oral candidiasis requiring antifungal treatment.

Systemic Corticosteroids

Drugs: Prednisone (oral), methylprednisolone (IV)

Uses: Acute asthma exacerbations, severe COPD exacerbations. Short bursts (5-10 days) or long-term for severe disease.

Adverse Effects (with prolonged use):

- Hyperglycemia—monitor blood glucose
- Immunosuppression—increased infection risk
- Osteoporosis—calcium, vitamin D, weight-bearing exercise
- Adrenal suppression—never stop abruptly after prolonged use
- Weight gain, fluid retention, mood changes, insomnia
- GI upset—take with food; may need PPI

Clinical Pearl: For short bursts (< 2 weeks), can stop without tapering. Longer courses require gradual taper to prevent adrenal crisis.

Leukotriene Modifiers

Drugs: Montelukast (Singulair), zafirlukast (Accolate), zileuton (Zyflo)

Mechanism: Block leukotriene receptors or synthesis → decrease inflammation, bronchoconstriction, mucus

Uses: Maintenance therapy for mild persistent asthma, allergic rhinitis, exercise-induced bronchospasm

Nursing Considerations:

- Montelukast: Take in evening (once daily)
- Zafirlukast: Take on empty stomach
- Zileuton: Monitor LFTs (hepatotoxicity)
- Not for acute bronchospasm

BLACK BOX WARNING (Montelukast): Serious neuropsychiatric events including agitation, depression, suicidal thoughts. Monitor mood changes.

Clinical Pearl: Montelukast is oral and once-daily—good option for patients who struggle with inhaler technique.

Mast Cell Stabilizers

Drug: Cromolyn sodium (Intal)

Mechanism: Prevents mast cell degranulation → prevents histamine release

Uses: Prophylaxis for exercise-induced bronchospasm, allergic asthma. Must be used BEFORE exposure.

Notes: Very safe but less effective than ICS. Rarely used now. Takes 2-4 weeks for full effect.

3.5 Combination Inhalers

Many patients benefit from combination products for convenience and compliance:

- Advair (fluticasone + salmeterol): ICS + LABA
- Symbicort (budesonide + formoterol): ICS + LABA
- Breo Ellipta (fluticasone + vilanterol): ICS + LABA, once daily
- Combivent (ipratropium + albuterol): Anticholinergic + SABA
- Trelegy Ellipta (fluticasone + umeclidinium + vilanterol): ICS + LAMA + LABA, once daily

Clinical Pearl: Combination inhalers improve adherence but patients must still understand each component's purpose.

3.6 Mucolytics and Expectorants

Mucolytics

Drug: Acetylcysteine (Mucomyst)

Mechanism: Breaks disulfide bonds in mucus → thins secretions

Uses: Cystic fibrosis, thick mucus conditions. Also antidote for ACETAMINOPHEN OVERDOSE.

Administration: Nebulized or oral (for acetaminophen overdose)

Adverse Effects: Bronchospasm (give bronchodilator first), unpleasant odor ("rotten eggs"), nausea

Expectorants

Drug: Guaifenesin (Mucinex, Robitussin)

Mechanism: Increases respiratory tract secretions → thins mucus → easier expectoration

Uses: Productive cough with thick mucus

Nursing Considerations: Encourage increased fluid intake (at least 8 glasses/day) to help thin secretions.

3.7 Antitussives

Opioid Antitussives: Codeine, hydrocodone. Suppress cough reflex centrally. Controlled substances. Cause sedation, constipation.

Non-Opioid Antitussives: Dextromethorphan (DM). Found in many OTC products (Robitussin DM, Delsym).

Nursing Considerations:

- Do not suppress productive cough (need to clear secretions)
- Use for dry, non-productive cough interfering with sleep
- Dextromethorphan: Avoid in patients on MAOIs (serotonin syndrome risk)

Clinical Pearl: Check combination products for multiple active ingredients—patients may inadvertently double-dose.

3.8 Antihistamines and Decongestants

Antihistamines

First-Generation (Sedating): Diphenhydramine (Benadryl), chlorpheniramine

- Cross blood-brain barrier → sedation, anticholinergic effects
- Adverse effects: Drowsiness, dry mouth, urinary retention, constipation, blurred vision
- Avoid in elderly (Beers Criteria), glaucoma, BPH

Second-Generation (Non-Sedating): Loratadine (Claritin), cetirizine (Zyrtec), fexofenadine (Allegra)

- Do not cross blood-brain barrier as readily → less sedation
- Preferred for allergic rhinitis

Intranasal: Azelastine (Astelin)—may cause drowsiness despite local application

Decongestants

Oral: Pseudoephedrine (Sudafed)

Mechanism: Alpha-adrenergic agonist → vasoconstriction → decreased nasal congestion

Adverse Effects: Increased HR, increased BP, insomnia, nervousness, urinary retention

Contraindications: Uncontrolled hypertension, severe CAD, MAOI use within 14 days

Nursing Considerations: Behind pharmacy counter (not prescription) due to use in methamphetamine production.

Topical (Nasal Sprays): Oxymetazoline (Afrin), phenylephrine

IMPORTANT: Limit use to 3-5 days maximum to prevent REBOUND CONGESTION (rhinitis medicamentosa).

Clinical Pearl: Ask hypertensive patients about decongestant use—many don't realize OTC products affect blood pressure.

3.9 Inhaler Devices and Administration

Proper inhaler technique is critical for medication effectiveness:

Metered-Dose Inhaler (MDI)

- Shake well before each use
- Exhale completely away from inhaler
- Place mouthpiece in mouth, seal lips
- Begin slow, deep inhalation while pressing canister
- Hold breath for 10 seconds if possible
- Wait 1 minute between puffs
- Use spacer device to improve delivery

Dry Powder Inhaler (DPI)

- Do NOT shake
- Exhale away from device (moisture affects powder)
- Inhale quickly and deeply (need sufficient inspiratory force)
- Hold breath for 10 seconds
- No spacer needed

Examples: Diskus, HandiHaler, Ellipta

Nebulizer

- Sit upright for best delivery
- Breathe normally through mouthpiece
- Continue until mist stops (5-15 minutes)
- Clean equipment after each use

Clinical Pearl: Have patients demonstrate technique at each visit—studies show up to 90% use inhalers incorrectly.

3.10 Asthma Management: Stepwise Approach

Asthma therapy follows a stepwise approach based on symptom control:

Step 1 (Intermittent): SABA as needed only

Step 2 (Mild Persistent): Low-dose ICS daily + SABA PRN

Step 3 (Moderate Persistent): Low-dose ICS + LABA, or medium-dose ICS

Step 4 (Moderate-Severe): Medium-dose ICS + LABA

Step 5 (Severe): High-dose ICS + LABA, consider biologics

Step 6: Add oral corticosteroids

Key principles: Step UP if not controlled. Step DOWN if well-controlled for 3 months.

3.11 COPD Management

COPD treatment differs from asthma:

- Bronchodilators are primary therapy (not ICS alone)
- Long-acting anticholinergics (tiotropium) often first-line
- ICS added for frequent exacerbations, usually with LABA
- Smoking cessation is MOST important intervention
- Pulmonary rehabilitation improves function
- Oxygen therapy for hypoxemia ($SpO_2 < 88\%$)

3.12 Chapter Summary

- SABAs (albuterol): Rescue medication for acute symptoms. Tremor, tachycardia common.
- LABAs: Maintenance only. BLACK BOX: Must use with ICS in asthma.
- Inhaled corticosteroids: First-line maintenance for asthma. RINSE MOUTH to prevent thrush.
- Anticholinergics: First-line for COPD. Dry mouth common. Caution in glaucoma, BPH.
- Theophylline: Narrow therapeutic index. Monitor levels. Many drug interactions.
- Nasal decongestants: Limit to 3-5 days to prevent rebound congestion.
- Proper inhaler technique is essential—have patients demonstrate.

3.13 Practice Questions

Directions: Select the best answer for each question.

1. A patient with asthma uses albuterol 4-5 times daily. The nurse should:

A. Reassure that this is appropriate rescue use

B. Recognize that asthma is not well controlled

C. Recommend switching to a long-acting bronchodilator

D. Suggest using albuterol only at bedtime

2. A patient prescribed fluticasone (Flovent) asks why they must rinse their mouth after use. The nurse explains:

A. To improve the taste of the medication

B. To prevent oral candidiasis

C. To increase absorption of the medication

D. To prevent staining of the teeth

3. Which medication should NEVER be used alone for asthma maintenance?

A. Fluticasone (Flovent)

B. Montelukast (Singulair)

C. Salmeterol (Serevent)

D. Budesonide (Pulmicort)

4. A patient uses both albuterol and fluticasone inhalers. The nurse teaches to:

A. Use fluticasone first, then albuterol

B. Use albuterol first, wait 5 minutes, then use fluticasone

C. Alternate days between the two medications

D. Mix both medications in a nebulizer

5. Which adverse effect is most commonly associated with inhaled anticholinergics?

A. Tachycardia

B. Dry mouth

C. Tremor

D. Hyperglycemia

6. A patient on theophylline should avoid:

A. Dairy products

B. Caffeine

C. Green leafy vegetables

D. Grapefruit juice

7. A patient using oxymetazoline (Afrin) nasal spray for 2 weeks reports worsening congestion. This is likely:

A. An allergic reaction

B. Rebound congestion

C. Medication tolerance

D. Incorrect administration technique

8. The nurse should question which order for a patient with uncontrolled hypertension?

A. Loratadine (Claritin)

B. Guaifenesin (Mucinex)

C. Pseudoephedrine (Sudafed)

D. Diphenhydramine (Benadryl)

9. When teaching a patient to use a dry powder inhaler, the nurse instructs to:

A. Shake vigorously before each use

B. Inhale slowly and steadily

C. Exhale into the device before inhaling

D. Inhale quickly and deeply

10. A patient with COPD is prescribed tiotropium (Spiriva). The nurse teaches:

A. This is a rescue inhaler for acute symptoms

B. Swallow the capsule whole with water

C. Use the HandiHaler device to inhale the powder

D. Expect immediate relief of symptoms

11. Acetylcysteine (Mucomyst) is also used as an antidote for:

A. Opioid overdose

B. Benzodiazepine overdose

C. Acetaminophen overdose

D. Aspirin overdose

12. Which statement indicates the patient understands montelukast (Singulair) therapy?

A. I will take this medication when I have an asthma attack

B. I should take this medication every evening

C. I can stop this medication when I feel better

D. This medication will work immediately

13. First-generation antihistamines like diphenhydramine should be avoided in older adults because:

A. They are not effective in older adults

B. They cause anticholinergic effects

C. They interact with all blood pressure medications

D. They must be given by injection

14. A patient using an MDI with a spacer demonstrates proper technique by:

A. Pressing the canister before starting to inhale

B. Holding breath for 2 seconds after inhalation

C. Shaking the inhaler and pressing while inhaling slowly

D. Breathing out through the spacer after inhalation

15. For a patient with persistent asthma not controlled on low-dose ICS, the next step would be:

A. Add oral prednisone daily

B. Increase SABA to scheduled dosing

C. Add a LABA to the regimen

D. Discontinue ICS and start theophylline

16. A patient prescribed prednisone 40 mg daily for 10 days for an asthma exacerbation asks about stopping the medication. The nurse responds:

A. You can stop abruptly after a short course like this

B. You must taper this medication over several weeks

C. You should never stop taking prednisone

D. You should only take it when you have symptoms

17. Which patient should the nurse assess for potential medication interaction with dextromethorphan?

A. Patient taking lisinopril

B. Patient taking phenelzine (an MAOI)

C. Patient taking atorvastatin

D. Patient taking metformin

18. A patient with newly diagnosed asthma should understand that inhaled corticosteroids:

A. Provide immediate relief of acute symptoms

B. Should be used daily even when feeling well

C. Can be stopped once symptoms improve

D. Work by relaxing bronchial smooth muscle

19. The most important intervention for a patient with COPD who continues to smoke is:

A. Increasing the dose of bronchodilators

B. Adding inhaled corticosteroids

C. Smoking cessation counseling and support

D. Starting prophylactic antibiotics

20. A patient reports white patches in their mouth after starting an inhaled corticosteroid. The nurse should:

A. Reassure that this is a harmless side effect

B. Recognize this as oral candidiasis requiring treatment

C. Discontinue the inhaled corticosteroid immediately

D. Recommend more frequent use of the medication

CHAPTER 4

Nervous System Medications

4.1 Learning Objectives

By the end of this chapter, you will be able to:

- Differentiate between the major classes of antidepressants and their mechanisms
- Identify the signs and symptoms of serotonin syndrome
- Explain the nursing considerations for antipsychotic medications
- Describe the therapeutic uses and monitoring parameters for mood stabilizers
- Recognize adverse effects of CNS depressants requiring intervention
- Apply safety principles for opioid administration
- Educate patients about antiepileptic drug therapy

4.2 Overview of CNS Pharmacology

The nervous system is divided into the central nervous system (CNS) and peripheral nervous system. CNS medications affect neurotransmitters including serotonin, norepinephrine, dopamine, GABA, and acetylcholine. This chapter covers medications for depression, anxiety, psychosis, seizures, pain, and neurodegenerative disorders.

4.3 Antidepressants

Selective Serotonin Reuptake Inhibitors (SSRIs)

Drugs: Fluoxetine (Prozac), sertraline (Zoloft), paroxetine (Paxil), citalopram (Celexa), escitalopram (Lexapro)

Mechanism: Block serotonin reuptake → increased serotonin in synapse

Uses: Depression (first-line), anxiety disorders, OCD, PTSD, panic disorder

Onset: 2-4 weeks for full therapeutic effect. Patients must be educated about this delay.

Adverse Effects:

- Sexual dysfunction (decreased libido, anorgasmia)—common reason for nonadherence
- GI effects (nausea, diarrhea)—usually improve over time

- CNS effects (headache, insomnia, anxiety initially)
- Weight changes
- Increased bleeding risk (especially with anticoagulants/NSAIDs)

BLACK BOX WARNING: Increased risk of suicidal thinking in children, adolescents, and young adults (< 25 years). Monitor closely, especially during first weeks.

Nursing Considerations:

- Takes 2-4 weeks for effect—encourage adherence
- Do not discontinue abruptly (withdrawal symptoms)
- Monitor for suicidal ideation, especially early in treatment
- Assess for serotonin syndrome if combined with other serotonergic drugs

Clinical Pearl: Fluoxetine has the longest half-life—less withdrawal risk but longer washout needed before switching.

Serotonin-Norepinephrine Reuptake Inhibitors (SNRIs)

Drugs: Venlafaxine (Effexor), duloxetine (Cymbalta), desvenlafaxine (Pristiq)

Mechanism: Block reuptake of both serotonin and norepinephrine

Uses: Depression, anxiety, neuropathic pain (duloxetine), fibromyalgia

Adverse Effects: Similar to SSRIs plus increased blood pressure (norepinephrine effect), especially venlafaxine at higher doses

Nursing Considerations: Monitor blood pressure. Same BLACK BOX WARNING as SSRIs.

Tricyclic Antidepressants (TCAs)

Drugs: Amitriptyline (Elavil), nortriptyline (Pamelor), imipramine (Tofranil)

Mechanism: Block reuptake of serotonin and norepinephrine; also block histamine, acetylcholine receptors

Uses: Depression (second-line), neuropathic pain, migraine prophylaxis, insomnia

Adverse Effects (Anticholinergic): Dry mouth, constipation, urinary retention, blurred vision, tachycardia

Cardiac Effects: QT prolongation, arrhythmias. Obtain baseline ECG.

Other: Sedation, orthostatic hypotension, weight gain

TOXICITY: TCAs are dangerous in overdose—cardiac arrhythmias, seizures, death. Not first-line due to safety concerns.

Clinical Pearl: Teach "anticholinergic effects" with memory aid: Can't see, can't pee, can't spit, can't... (defecate).

Monoamine Oxidase Inhibitors (MAOIs)

Drugs: Phenelzine (Nardil), tranylcypromine (Parnate), selegiline (EMSAM patch)

Mechanism: Inhibit MAO enzyme → increased serotonin, norepinephrine, dopamine

Uses: Treatment-resistant depression. Rarely used due to interactions.

CRITICAL INTERACTION - TYRAMINE: Foods high in tyramine can cause HYPERTENSIVE CRISIS.

- Avoid: Aged cheeses, cured meats, tap beer, soy sauce, sauerkraut, fermented foods
- Symptoms: Severe headache, hypertension, nausea, vomiting—can lead to stroke

Drug Interactions: Do NOT combine with SSRIs, SNRIs, meperidine, dextromethorphan—SEROTONIN SYNDROME risk. Requires 2-week washout.

Serotonin Syndrome

Cause: Excessive serotonergic activity, usually from drug combinations

Classic Triad:

- Mental status changes (agitation, confusion)
- Autonomic instability (hyperthermia, tachycardia, diaphoresis, hypertension)
- Neuromuscular abnormalities (tremor, hyperreflexia, clonus, rigidity)

Treatment: Stop offending drugs, supportive care, benzodiazepines for agitation, cyproheptadine (serotonin antagonist) in severe cases.

Clinical Pearl: Serotonin syndrome can occur within hours. Differentiate from neuroleptic malignant syndrome (NMS)—SS has hyperreflexia/clonus; NMS has "lead pipe" rigidity.

4.4 Anxiolytics and Sedative-Hypnotics

Benzodiazepines

Drugs: Lorazepam (Ativan), diazepam (Valium), alprazolam (Xanax), midazolam (Versed), clonazepam (Klonopin)

Mechanism: Enhance GABA activity → CNS depression

Uses: Anxiety, insomnia, seizures, alcohol withdrawal, procedural sedation, muscle relaxation

Adverse Effects: Sedation, confusion, respiratory depression, ataxia, amnesia, dependence

HIGH-ALERT: CNS depression potentiated by opioids, alcohol, other sedatives. BLACK BOX WARNING for concurrent opioid use.

Nursing Considerations:

- Monitor respiratory status, especially with opioids
- Fall precautions (sedation, ataxia)
- Avoid abrupt discontinuation after prolonged use (seizures, withdrawal)
- Use lower doses in elderly (Beers Criteria)

Antidote: Flumazenil—use cautiously (can precipitate seizures in chronic users)

Clinical Pearl: Lorazepam (Ativan) preferred in liver disease—no active metabolites.

Non-Benzodiazepine Hypnotics (Z-drugs)

Drugs: Zolpidem (Ambien), eszopiclone (Lunesta), zaleplon (Sonata)

Uses: Short-term insomnia treatment

Adverse Effects: Complex sleep behaviors (sleepwalking, sleep-driving, sleep-eating), next-day impairment, amnesia

BLACK BOX WARNING: Complex sleep behaviors can cause serious injury. Discontinue if occurs.

Nursing Considerations: Take immediately before bed. Do not take unless able to get 7-8 hours sleep. Lower dose for women.

Buspirone (BuSpar)

Mechanism: Serotonin receptor partial agonist

Uses: Generalized anxiety disorder (GAD)

Advantages: No sedation, no dependence, no interaction with alcohol

Disadvantage: Takes 2-4 weeks for effect (not for acute anxiety)

Clinical Pearl: Good option for patients with history of substance abuse (no dependence potential).

4.5 Antipsychotics

First-Generation (Typical) Antipsychotics

Drugs: Haloperidol (Haldol), chlorpromazine (Thorazine), fluphenazine

Mechanism: Block dopamine D2 receptors

Uses: Schizophrenia, acute psychosis, severe agitation, Tourette syndrome

Adverse Effects:

Extrapyramidal Symptoms (EPS):

- Acute dystonia (muscle spasms, torticollis)—treat with benztropine or diphenhydramine
- Akathisia (restlessness, inability to sit still)
- Parkinsonism (bradykinesia, rigidity, tremor)
- Tardive dyskinesia (late-onset involuntary movements, often irreversible)—assess with AIMS scale

Neuroleptic Malignant Syndrome (NMS): Life-threatening. Hyperthermia, severe rigidity ("lead pipe"), altered consciousness, autonomic instability. Stop drug immediately. Supportive care, dantrolene.

Other Effects: Sedation, anticholinergic effects, orthostatic hypotension, QT prolongation, hyperprolactinemia (galactorrhea, amenorrhea)

Second-Generation (Atypical) Antipsychotics

Drugs: Risperidone (Risperdal), olanzapine (Zyprexa), quetiapine (Seroquel), aripiprazole (Abilify), clozapine (Clozaril), ziprasidone (Geodon)

Mechanism: Block dopamine and serotonin receptors

Uses: Schizophrenia, bipolar disorder, depression augmentation, irritability in autism

Advantages: Lower EPS risk than first-generation (but still possible)

Metabolic Adverse Effects:

- Weight gain (especially olanzapine, clozapine)
- Hyperglycemia, new-onset diabetes
- Hyperlipidemia

Monitoring: Baseline and periodic: Weight, fasting glucose, lipid panel, blood pressure

CLOZAPINE SPECIAL CONSIDERATIONS:

- Most effective for treatment-resistant schizophrenia
- AGRANULOCYTOSIS risk—requires weekly to monthly WBC/ANC monitoring (REMS program)
- Also causes severe constipation, seizures, myocarditis

BLACK BOX WARNING (All Antipsychotics): Increased mortality in elderly with dementia-related psychosis.

4.6 Mood Stabilizers

Lithium

Uses: Bipolar disorder (first-line for mania prophylaxis)

NARROW THERAPEUTIC INDEX: Therapeutic range 0.6-1.2 mEq/L. Toxicity common.

Adverse Effects:

- GI (nausea, diarrhea)
- Fine tremor
- Polyuria, polydipsia (nephrogenic diabetes insipidus)
- Hypothyroidism (monitor thyroid function)
- Weight gain

Lithium Toxicity Signs:

- Mild (1.5-2.0): Coarse tremor, GI distress, muscle weakness
- Moderate (2.0-2.5): Confusion, ataxia, slurred speech
- Severe (>2.5): Seizures, coma, death

Nursing Considerations:

- Monitor lithium levels (draw 12 hours after last dose)
- Monitor renal function, thyroid function
- Maintain adequate sodium and fluid intake (dehydration increases levels)
- Avoid NSAIDs, ACE inhibitors, thiazide diuretics (increase lithium levels)

Clinical Pearl: Teach patients: Maintain consistent salt/fluid intake. Avoid dehydration. Report vomiting/diarrhea (can increase levels quickly).

Anticonvulsants as Mood Stabilizers

Valproic Acid (Depakote): Bipolar disorder, seizures, migraine prophylaxis. Monitor LFTs, CBC. Teratogenic—avoid in pregnancy. Weight gain, hair loss, tremor.

Carbamazepine (Tegretol): Bipolar disorder, seizures, trigeminal neuralgia. Induces own metabolism. Monitor CBC (aplastic anemia risk). Many drug interactions.

Lamotrigine (Lamictal): Bipolar depression. STEVENS-JOHNSON SYNDROME risk—titrate slowly. Stop immediately if rash develops.

4.7 Antiepileptic Drugs (AEDs)

Many AEDs have multiple mechanisms and uses beyond seizures.

Key Antiepileptic Drugs

Phenytoin (Dilantin):

- Uses: Tonic-clonic seizures, status epilepticus
- NARROW THERAPEUTIC INDEX: 10-20 mcg/mL

- Zero-order kinetics—small dose changes cause large level changes
- Adverse effects: Gingival hyperplasia, hirsutism, ataxia, nystagmus, osteoporosis
- IV administration: Give slowly (no faster than 50 mg/min)—cardiac arrhythmias, hypotension
- Many drug interactions (CYP450 inducer)

Levetiracetam (Keppra):

- Broad-spectrum AED
- Few drug interactions (not metabolized by CYP450)
- May cause behavioral changes, irritability

Phenobarbital:

- Oldest AED, still used
- Barbiturate—CNS depression, sedation
- CYP450 inducer (many interactions)

General AED Principles:

- Never discontinue abruptly (risk of status epilepticus)
- Many are teratogenic—counsel women of childbearing age
- Monitor drug levels for narrow TI drugs
- Folic acid supplementation often recommended

4.8 Opioid Analgesics

Opioid Agonists

Drugs: Morphine, hydromorphone (Dilaudid), fentanyl, oxycodone, hydrocodone, codeine, methadone

Mechanism: Bind to mu opioid receptors → analgesia, euphoria, respiratory depression

Uses: Moderate to severe pain, cough suppression (codeine), anesthesia (fentanyl)

HIGH-ALERT MEDICATION: Opioids are among the highest-risk drugs in hospitals.

Adverse Effects:

- Respiratory depression (most serious)—monitor RR, SpO2, sedation level
- Sedation
- Constipation (tolerance does NOT develop—always address)
- Nausea, vomiting
- Urinary retention

- Pruritus (histamine release)
- Hypotension

Nursing Considerations:

- Assess pain before and after administration
- Monitor respiratory rate—hold if RR < 12
- Have naloxone available
- Implement bowel regimen (stool softener, laxative)
- Fall precautions
- Assess for signs of overdose: pinpoint pupils, respiratory depression, decreased LOC

Antidote: Naloxone (Narcan)—opioid antagonist. May need repeated doses (shorter half-life than most opioids).

Clinical Pearl: Meperidine (Demerol) is avoided due to toxic metabolite (normeperidine) causing seizures, especially in renal impairment.

Opioid Agonist-Antagonists

Drugs: Buprenorphine (Subutex, Suboxone), nalbuphine (Nubain), butorphanol (Stadol)

Properties: Partial agonists—ceiling effect on respiratory depression. Can precipitate withdrawal in opioid-dependent patients.

Buprenorphine: Used for opioid use disorder treatment (often combined with naloxone as Suboxone).

4.9 Non-Opioid Analgesics

Acetaminophen (Tylenol)

Uses: Mild to moderate pain, fever reduction

Max Dose: 3-4 g/day in healthy adults; 2 g/day with liver disease or alcohol use

HEPATOTOXICITY: Leading cause of acute liver failure. Found in many combination products—patients may unknowingly exceed limits.

Antidote: Acetylcysteine (Mucomyst)—most effective within 8 hours of overdose

Clinical Pearl: Always ask about OTC medications and combination products containing acetaminophen.

NSAIDs

Drugs: Ibuprofen (Advil, Motrin), naproxen (Aleve), ketorolac (Toradol), celecoxib (Celebrex)

Mechanism: Inhibit cyclooxygenase (COX) → decreased prostaglandins

Uses: Pain, inflammation, fever

Adverse Effects:

- GI (ulcers, bleeding)—take with food
- Renal impairment—avoid in kidney disease
- Cardiovascular risk (increased MI, stroke)—BLACK BOX WARNING
- Platelet inhibition (increased bleeding)

Contraindications: Avoid before surgery, with anticoagulants, in renal disease, in GI bleeding history, third trimester pregnancy

Clinical Pearl: Ketorolac (Toradol) is limited to 5 days due to high GI bleeding risk.

4.10 Drugs for Parkinson's Disease

Pathophysiology: Loss of dopaminergic neurons in substantia nigra → dopamine/acetylcholine imbalance

Levodopa/Carbidopa (Sinemet):

- Most effective treatment—levodopa converted to dopamine in brain
- Carbidopa prevents peripheral conversion
- Adverse effects: Nausea, orthostatic hypotension, dyskinesias (involuntary movements), "on-off" phenomenon
- Avoid high-protein meals (compete for absorption)
- Avoid with MAOIs

Dopamine Agonists: Pramipexole (Mirapex), ropinirole (Requip). Can cause sleep attacks, impulse control disorders.

Anticholinergics: Benztropine (Cogentin). Used for tremor and drug-induced EPS. Avoid in elderly.

4.11 Drugs for Alzheimer's Disease

Cholinesterase Inhibitors: Donepezil (Aricept), rivastigmine (Exelon), galantamine (Razadyne)

- Increase acetylcholine by inhibiting breakdown
- Modest improvement in cognition; do not cure or halt progression
- Adverse effects: GI (nausea, diarrhea), bradycardia

NMDA Antagonist: Memantine (Namenda). Used in moderate-severe Alzheimer's. May combine with cholinesterase inhibitor.

4.12 Chapter Summary

- SSRIs: First-line for depression. 2-4 weeks onset. BLACK BOX for suicidality in youth. Watch for serotonin syndrome.
- MAOIs: Tyramine restriction essential—avoid aged cheese, cured meats. Hypertensive crisis risk.
- Benzodiazepines: CNS depression with opioids. Avoid abrupt discontinuation. Flumazenil is antidote.
- Antipsychotics: First-gen causes EPS. Second-gen causes metabolic syndrome. Both can cause NMS.
- Lithium: Narrow TI (0.6-1.2). Monitor levels, renal, thyroid. Maintain hydration and sodium.
- Opioids: HIGH-ALERT. Monitor RR. Constipation always addressed. Naloxone is antidote.
- Acetaminophen: Max 3-4 g/day. Hepatotoxicity risk. Antidote is acetylcysteine.

4.13 Practice Questions

Directions: Select the best answer for each question.

1. A patient starting fluoxetine (Prozac) asks when they will feel better. The nurse responds:

A. You should feel better within 24-48 hours

B. It typically takes 2-4 weeks to notice improvement

C. The medication works immediately but takes time to build up

D. You will feel worse for the first month

2. A patient taking phenelzine (Nardil) should avoid which food?

A. Fresh chicken

B. White bread

C. Aged cheese

D. Cooked vegetables

3. A patient on multiple serotonergic medications develops agitation, hyperthermia, tremor, and hyperreflexia. The nurse suspects:

A. Neuroleptic malignant syndrome

B. Serotonin syndrome

C. Anticholinergic toxicity

D. Opioid withdrawal

4. Which finding would cause the nurse to hold a scheduled dose of lorazepam?

A. Heart rate of 88 bpm

B. Respiratory rate of 10 breaths/min

C. Blood pressure of 128/78 mmHg

D. Temperature of 98.8°F

5. A patient on haloperidol develops severe muscle rigidity, hyperthermia, and altered consciousness. The priority action is:

A. Administer benztropine

B. Continue haloperidol and monitor

C. Stop haloperidol and notify provider immediately

D. Give acetaminophen for fever

6. A patient taking lithium has a level of 1.8 mEq/L with confusion and ataxia. The nurse should:

A. Continue the current dose

B. Recognize this as lithium toxicity

C. Increase fluid intake and repeat the level

D. Give the next dose as scheduled

7. Which instruction is most important for a patient taking lithium?

A. Avoid all caffeine intake

B. Maintain consistent salt and fluid intake

C. Take the medication on an empty stomach

D. Avoid exposure to sunlight

8. A patient taking clozapine should be monitored for:

A. Renal function weekly

B. White blood cell count regularly

C. Thyroid function monthly

D. Potassium levels daily

9. The nurse should question an order for meperidine (Demerol) in a patient with:

A. Mild liver disease

B. Chronic kidney disease

C. Controlled hypertension

D. Type 2 diabetes

10. A patient receiving morphine has a respiratory rate of 8 and is difficult to arouse. The priority intervention is:

A. Administer naloxone

B. Stimulate the patient and encourage deep breathing

C. Document findings and continue monitoring

D. Hold the next scheduled dose

11. A patient taking phenytoin (Dilantin) should be taught to:

A. Expect drowsiness for the first week

B. Practice good oral hygiene to prevent gum overgrowth

C. Take the medication with antacids

D. Stop the medication if seizure-free for 6 months

12. Which patient statement indicates understanding of SSRI therapy?

A. I can stop this medication once I feel better

B. I should avoid aged cheeses while taking this

C. I may experience sexual side effects

D. This medication will work within a few hours

13. A patient on opioid therapy has not had a bowel movement in 4 days. The nurse should:

A. Recognize this is an expected effect that will resolve

B. Administer prescribed laxatives and increase fluids

C. Hold the opioid until bowel function returns

D. Reassure that constipation is not serious

14. A patient taking carbamazepine (Tegretol) should report which finding immediately?

A. Mild drowsiness

B. Dry mouth

C. Sore throat and fever

D. Slight dizziness when standing

15. The antidote for benzodiazepine overdose is:

A. Naloxone

B. Flumazenil

C. Acetylcysteine

D. Protamine sulfate

16. A patient asks why they cannot drink alcohol while taking alprazolam. The nurse explains:

A. Alcohol decreases the effectiveness of the medication

B. The combination increases CNS depression and can be fatal

C. Alcohol causes the medication to be excreted faster

D. There is no interaction between alcohol and alprazolam

17. A patient taking olanzapine (Zyprexa) should be monitored for:

A. Hypothyroidism

B. Weight gain and hyperglycemia

C. Decreased white blood cell count

D. Pulmonary toxicity

18. An elderly patient with dementia is prescribed quetiapine. The nurse should be aware that:

A. This is the safest antipsychotic for elderly patients

B. There is increased risk of mortality in this population

C. Dementia patients respond better to antipsychotics

D. Quetiapine does not cause sedation in elderly

19. A patient on levodopa/carbidopa should avoid:

A. High-protein meals taken with the medication

B. Fresh fruits and vegetables

C. Whole grain bread

D. Dairy products in the evening

20. Which assessment finding indicates acetaminophen toxicity?

A. Tinnitus and dizziness

B. Right upper quadrant pain and jaundice

C. Decreased urine output and edema

D. Tachycardia and hypertension

CHAPTER 5

Endocrine Medications

5.1 Learning Objectives

By the end of this chapter, you will be able to:

- Differentiate between types of insulin and their onset, peak, and duration
- Identify the mechanisms and nursing considerations for oral antidiabetic agents
- Explain the management of thyroid disorders with appropriate medications
- Recognize the adverse effects of corticosteroids requiring intervention
- Apply safety principles for insulin administration
- Describe the treatment of adrenal disorders
- Educate patients about diabetes medication management and hypoglycemia

5.2 Overview of Endocrine Pharmacology

The endocrine system regulates metabolism, growth, reproduction, and homeostasis through hormones. Endocrine medications either replace deficient hormones, suppress excess hormone production, or modify hormone action. This chapter covers diabetes medications, thyroid drugs, corticosteroids, and other hormonal therapies.

5.3 Diabetes Medications: Insulin

HIGH-ALERT MEDICATION: Insulin is one of the most dangerous medications due to hypoglycemia risk. Always verify dose with another nurse.

Types of Insulin

Rapid-Acting:

- Lispro (Humalog), aspart (NovoLog), glulisine (Apidra)
- Onset: 10-15 minutes; Peak: 1-2 hours; Duration: 3-5 hours
- Give immediately before meals (within 15 minutes)
- Clear appearance

Short-Acting (Regular):

- Regular insulin (Humulin R, Novolin R)
- Onset: 30-60 minutes; Peak: 2-4 hours; Duration: 5-8 hours
- Give 30 minutes before meals
- Clear appearance; ONLY insulin for IV use

Intermediate-Acting:

- NPH (Humulin N, Novolin N)
- Onset: 1-2 hours; Peak: 4-12 hours; Duration: 18-24 hours
- Cloudy appearance—must roll gently to mix (do not shake)
- Usually given once or twice daily

Long-Acting:

- Glargine (Lantus, Basaglar), detemir (Levemir), degludec (Tresiba)
- Onset: 1-2 hours; No peak (relatively peakless); Duration: 24+ hours
- Clear appearance; give once daily at same time
- Do NOT mix with other insulins

Clinical Pearl: "Clear before cloudy"—when mixing regular and NPH in same syringe, draw up clear (regular) first to prevent contamination.

Insulin Administration

- Rotate injection sites (abdomen absorbs fastest, then arms, thighs, buttocks)
- Do not inject into same site repeatedly (lipodystrophy)
- Store unopened insulin in refrigerator; opened vials at room temperature for 28 days
- Verify dose with another nurse (high-alert medication)
- Use insulin syringes or insulin pens—never use TB syringes

Hypoglycemia

Signs/Symptoms: Shakiness, sweating, tachycardia, confusion, irritability, hunger, pallor

Treatment (Rule of 15):

- Give 15 g fast-acting carbohydrate (4 oz juice, glucose tablets)
- Recheck blood glucose in 15 minutes
- Repeat if still < 70 mg/dL
- Follow with protein/complex carb snack

Severe Hypoglycemia (unconscious): Glucagon IM/SubQ or IV dextrose (D50). Never give oral glucose to unconscious patient.

Hyperglycemia and DKA

DKA Signs: Hyperglycemia (>250), ketones, fruity breath, Kussmaul respirations, dehydration, altered mental status

Treatment: IV fluids, IV regular insulin, electrolyte replacement (especially potassium)

Clinical Pearl: In DKA, potassium shifts out of cells. Serum K+ may appear normal or high, but total body K+ is depleted. Replace K+ before it drops dangerously.

5.4 Oral Antidiabetic Agents

Biguanides

Drug: Metformin (Glucophage)—FIRST-LINE for Type 2 diabetes

Mechanism: Decreases hepatic glucose production, increases insulin sensitivity

Advantages: Weight neutral or weight loss, low hypoglycemia risk (when used alone), cardiovascular benefits

Adverse Effects: GI upset (diarrhea, nausea)—start low, take with food

SERIOUS: Lactic Acidosis (rare but potentially fatal)

- Risk factors: Renal impairment, liver disease, heart failure, hypoxia
- Contraindicated if eGFR < 30 mL/min
- Hold before and 48 hours after IV contrast procedures

Clinical Pearl: Metformin does not cause hypoglycemia when used alone—it doesn't increase insulin secretion.

Sulfonylureas

Drugs: Glipizide (Glucotrol), glyburide (DiaBeta), glimepiride (Amaryl)

Mechanism: Stimulate pancreatic beta cells to release insulin

Adverse Effects: HYPOGLYCEMIA (primary concern), weight gain

Nursing Considerations:

- Take 30 minutes before meals
- Teach hypoglycemia recognition and treatment
- Avoid alcohol (disulfiram-like reaction with some agents)
- Use caution in elderly and renal impairment

SGLT2 Inhibitors

Drugs: Canagliflozin (Invokana), dapagliflozin (Farxiga), empagliflozin (Jardiance)

Memory Tip: End in "-gliflozin"

Mechanism: Block glucose reabsorption in kidney → glucose excreted in urine

Benefits: Weight loss, BP reduction, cardiovascular and renal protection

Adverse Effects:

- Genital yeast infections (glucosuria promotes fungal growth)
- Urinary tract infections
- Polyuria, dehydration, hypotension
- Euglycemic DKA (DKA with near-normal glucose—can be missed!)

BLACK BOX (Canagliflozin): Increased risk of lower limb amputation

Clinical Pearl: SGLT2 inhibitors now used for heart failure and CKD even without diabetes.

GLP-1 Receptor Agonists

Drugs: Liraglutide (Victoza), semaglutide (Ozempic, Wegovy), dulaglutide (Trulicity), exenatide (Byetta)

Memory Tip: End in "-glutide"

Mechanism: Mimic incretin hormones → increase insulin secretion, decrease glucagon, slow gastric emptying

Administration: SubQ injection (most are weekly)

Benefits: Significant weight loss, cardiovascular protection

Adverse Effects: Nausea, vomiting (usually improves), injection site reactions

BLACK BOX WARNING: Thyroid C-cell tumors in rodents—contraindicated in patients with personal/family history of medullary thyroid cancer or MEN2

Clinical Pearl: Semaglutide (Wegovy/Ozempic) is now widely used for weight management.

DPP-4 Inhibitors

Drugs: Sitagliptin (Januvia), saxagliptin (Onglyza), linagliptin (Tradjenta)

Memory Tip: End in "-gliptin"

Mechanism: Inhibit DPP-4 enzyme → prolong incretin action → increase insulin, decrease glucagon

Advantages: Oral, weight neutral, low hypoglycemia risk

Adverse Effects: Upper respiratory infections, headache, pancreatitis (rare)

Thiazolidinediones (TZDs)

Drugs: Pioglitazone (Actos), rosiglitazone (Avandia)

Memory Tip: End in "-glitazone"

Mechanism: Increase insulin sensitivity in peripheral tissues

Adverse Effects: Weight gain, fluid retention, edema

BLACK BOX WARNING: Contraindicated in heart failure (fluid retention worsens HF)

Other Concerns: Increased fracture risk, bladder cancer risk (pioglitazone)

5.5 Thyroid Medications

Hypothyroidism Treatment

Drug: Levothyroxine (Synthroid, Levoxyl)—synthetic T4

Uses: Hypothyroidism, thyroid replacement after thyroidectomy

Administration:

- Take on EMPTY STOMACH, 30-60 minutes before breakfast
- Take at same time daily for consistent levels
- Separate from calcium, iron, antacids by 4 hours (decrease absorption)

Monitoring: TSH levels (goal: normalize TSH). Check 6-8 weeks after dose changes.

Adverse Effects (signs of excess/hyperthyroidism): Tachycardia, palpitations, weight loss, nervousness, insomnia, heat intolerance

Clinical Pearl: Start low in elderly and cardiac patients—excess thyroid hormone can precipitate angina or MI.

Hyperthyroidism Treatment

Thioamides:

- Methimazole (Tapazole)—preferred; once daily dosing
- Propylthiouracil (PTU)—preferred in first trimester pregnancy and thyroid storm

Mechanism: Inhibit thyroid hormone synthesis

Adverse Effects:

- Agranulocytosis (rare but serious)—report sore throat, fever immediately
- Hepatotoxicity (especially PTU)—BLACK BOX WARNING
- Rash, GI upset

Radioactive Iodine (I-131): Destroys thyroid tissue. Contraindicated in pregnancy. Patient is radioactive—isolation precautions needed.

Beta Blockers: Used for symptom control (tachycardia, tremor) while awaiting thioamide effect.

Thyroid Storm

Medical Emergency: Severe hyperthyroidism with fever, tachycardia, altered mental status, heart failure

Treatment: PTU (blocks synthesis AND conversion), beta blockers, corticosteroids, cooling measures, supportive care

5.6 Corticosteroids

Drugs: Prednisone, prednisolone, methylprednisolone, hydrocortisone, dexamethasone

Mechanism: Anti-inflammatory and immunosuppressive effects

Uses: Inflammatory conditions, autoimmune diseases, allergic reactions, asthma exacerbations, adrenal insufficiency replacement

Adverse Effects (with prolonged use)

Metabolic:

- Hyperglycemia (steroid-induced diabetes)—monitor blood glucose
- Weight gain, fluid retention, "moon face," "buffalo hump"
- Hypokalemia

Musculoskeletal:

- Osteoporosis—calcium, vitamin D, bisphosphonates for prevention
- Muscle weakness
- Growth suppression in children

Immune:

- Increased infection risk (immunosuppression)
- Masks signs of infection

GI: Peptic ulcer, GI bleeding—take with food; may need PPI

Other: Mood changes, insomnia, cataracts, thin skin, easy bruising

Critical Considerations

Adrenal Suppression: Long-term use suppresses HPA axis. NEVER stop abruptly—taper gradually to prevent adrenal crisis.

Adrenal Crisis: Life-threatening hypotension, hypoglycemia, altered consciousness. Give IV hydrocortisone.

Stress Dosing: Patients on chronic steroids need increased doses during illness, surgery, or trauma.

Clinical Pearl: Patients on long-term steroids should wear medical alert identification and carry emergency steroid information.

5.7 Adrenal Disorders

Adrenal Insufficiency (Addison's Disease)

Treatment: Hormone replacement with hydrocortisone (glucocorticoid) and fludrocortisone (mineralocorticoid)

Fludrocortisone: Replaces aldosterone—monitor for fluid retention, hypertension, hypokalemia

Patient Education: Lifelong therapy, stress dosing, medical alert bracelet

Cushing's Syndrome

Cause: Excess cortisol (often from exogenous steroids or pituitary adenoma)

Treatment: Depends on cause. If drug-induced, taper steroids. May need surgery or medications to suppress cortisol.

5.8 Pituitary Hormones

Growth Hormone

Drug: Somatropin (Genotropin, Humatrope)

Uses: Growth hormone deficiency in children and adults, Turner syndrome

Administration: SubQ injection, usually at bedtime (mimics physiologic secretion)

Antidiuretic Hormone (ADH)

Drug: Desmopressin (DDAVP)

Uses: Diabetes insipidus (central), nocturnal enuresis, von Willebrand disease

Adverse Effects: Water retention, hyponatremia—monitor fluid status and sodium

5.9 Bone and Calcium Disorders

Bisphosphonates

Drugs: Alendronate (Fosamax), risedronate (Actonel), ibandronate (Boniva), zoledronic acid (Reclast)

Mechanism: Inhibit osteoclast activity → decrease bone resorption

Uses: Osteoporosis prevention and treatment, Paget's disease

Administration (oral):

- Take first thing in morning on EMPTY stomach with FULL glass of water
- Remain UPRIGHT for 30-60 minutes (prevents esophageal irritation)
- Do not eat, drink, or take other medications for 30-60 minutes

Adverse Effects:

- Esophagitis, esophageal ulcers (if not taken properly)
- Osteonecrosis of the jaw (rare)—dental exam before starting
- Atypical femur fractures (with long-term use)

Clinical Pearl: Many patients are non-adherent due to complex administration. Weekly or monthly formulations may improve compliance.

Calcium and Vitamin D

Calcium Supplements: Calcium carbonate (take with food), calcium citrate (can take without food)

Vitamin D: Cholecalciferol (D3), ergocalciferol (D2). Essential for calcium absorption.

Nursing Considerations: Space calcium from other medications (decreases absorption of many drugs including levothyroxine, bisphosphonates, fluoroquinolones)

5.10 Sex Hormones

Estrogen/Progestin Therapy

Uses: Contraception, menopausal symptoms, hormone replacement

Contraindications: History of DVT/PE, stroke, breast cancer, liver disease, pregnancy, smoking > 35 years old

Adverse Effects: Increased clot risk (DVT, PE, stroke), breast tenderness, nausea, headache

Clinical Pearl: Teach patients to report leg pain, chest pain, severe headache, vision changes (signs of clot).

Testosterone

Uses: Male hypogonadism, delayed puberty

Adverse Effects: Polycythemia (increased RBCs), liver toxicity, mood changes, acne, gynecomastia

BLACK BOX WARNING: Secondary exposure risk—women and children can absorb testosterone from skin contact with application sites

5.11 Chapter Summary

- Insulin: HIGH-ALERT. Know onset/peak/duration. Rapid-acting before meals; long-acting once daily. Hypoglycemia is major risk.
- Metformin: First-line for T2DM. Hold for contrast. Lactic acidosis risk. Does not cause hypoglycemia alone.
- Sulfonylureas: Cause HYPOGLYCEMIA. Take before meals.
- SGLT2 inhibitors: Cause glucosuria, genital infections. Watch for euglycemic DKA.
- GLP-1 agonists: Weight loss, weekly injection. BLACK BOX for thyroid tumors.
- Levothyroxine: Empty stomach, separate from calcium/iron. Monitor TSH.
- Corticosteroids: NEVER stop abruptly (adrenal crisis). Monitor glucose, bones, infection.
- Bisphosphonates: Take upright with water. Risk of esophagitis, jaw osteonecrosis.

5.12 Practice Questions

Directions: Select the best answer for each question.

1. A patient receives NPH insulin at 7:00 AM. The nurse should monitor most closely for hypoglycemia at:

A. 8:00 AM

B. 12:00 PM (noon)

C. 6:00 PM

D. 10:00 PM

2. A patient taking metformin is scheduled for a CT scan with IV contrast. The nurse should:

A. Continue metformin as prescribed

B. Hold metformin before and for 48 hours after the procedure

C. Give metformin with extra fluids

D. Administer metformin after the procedure only

3. Which statement indicates a patient understands levothyroxine administration?

A. I will take this medication with my breakfast

B. I will take this medication on an empty stomach in the morning

C. I will take this medication with my calcium supplement

D. I will take this medication at bedtime with a snack

4. A patient on long-term prednisone is being discharged. Which instruction is most important?

A. Stop the medication when you feel better

B. Decrease the dose gradually as prescribed

C. Take the medication only when needed

D. Double the dose if you miss a dose

5. A diabetic patient experiences shakiness, sweating, and confusion. Blood glucose is 58 mg/dL. The priority intervention is:

A. Administer regular insulin

B. Give 4 oz of orange juice

C. Recheck blood glucose in 15 minutes

D. Call the healthcare provider

6. Which adverse effect is associated with SGLT2 inhibitors like canagliflozin?

A. Hypoglycemia when used alone

B. Weight gain

C. Genital yeast infections

D. Increased blood pressure

7. A patient taking glipizide should be taught to:

A. Take the medication at bedtime

B. Recognize and treat hypoglycemia symptoms

C. Expect significant weight loss

D. Avoid eating before taking the medication

8. Before administering the first dose of alendronate (Fosamax), the nurse should instruct the patient to:

A. Take the medication with orange juice

B. Remain upright for at least 30 minutes after taking

C. Crush the tablet if difficulty swallowing

D. Take the medication with a calcium supplement

9. A patient receiving methimazole for hyperthyroidism should report which symptom immediately?

A. Mild fatigue

B. Sore throat and fever

C. Slight weight gain

D. Dry skin

10. The nurse is preparing to mix regular and NPH insulin in the same syringe. The correct technique is:

A. Draw NPH first, then regular

B. Draw regular first, then NPH

C. Either order is acceptable

D. These insulins cannot be mixed

11. A patient with Type 2 diabetes asks why they are prescribed metformin instead of insulin. The nurse explains:

A. Metformin works faster than insulin

B. Metformin increases insulin sensitivity and is first-line therapy

C. Insulin is only for Type 1 diabetes

D. Metformin has no side effects

12. A patient on chronic corticosteroid therapy develops a respiratory infection. The nurse anticipates:

A. Decreasing the steroid dose

B. Increasing the steroid dose temporarily

C. Discontinuing the steroid immediately

D. No change in steroid therapy

13. Which insulin can be administered intravenously?

A. NPH (Humulin N)

B. Glargine (Lantus)

C. Regular (Humulin R)

D. Lispro (Humalog)

14. A patient taking liraglutide (Victoza) reports persistent nausea. The nurse should:

A. Discontinue the medication immediately

B. Explain this often improves with continued use

C. Administer an antiemetic with each dose

D. Switch to oral medication immediately

15. A patient receiving insulin glargine asks why it is given at bedtime. The nurse explains:

A. It works best when given at night

B. It has no peak and provides 24-hour coverage

C. It must be given when fasting

D. It causes less hypoglycemia at night

16. Which finding in a patient taking pioglitazone (Actos) requires immediate notification of the provider?

A. Mild headache

B. Weight gain of 2 pounds over a month

C. New onset shortness of breath and leg edema

D. Occasional mild nausea

17. A patient with Addison's disease should be taught to:

A. Decrease medication during times of stress

B. Wear a medical alert bracelet

C. Restrict sodium intake

D. Stop medication if feeling well

18. The nurse should question an order for GLP-1 agonist therapy in a patient with:

A. Type 2 diabetes

B. Obesity

C. Personal history of medullary thyroid cancer

D. Hypertension

19. A patient taking semaglutide for weight management asks about common side effects. The nurse includes:

A. Increased appetite

B. Nausea and vomiting

C. Hypoglycemia requiring frequent snacks

D. Significant hair loss

20. A diabetic patient is found unconscious. After confirming hypoglycemia, the priority action is:

A. Give oral glucose gel

B. Administer glucagon or IV dextrose

C. Wait for the patient to wake up

D. Administer regular insulin

CHAPTER 6

Gastrointestinal Medications

6.1 Learning Objectives

By the end of this chapter, you will be able to:

- Differentiate between classes of acid-reducing medications
- Identify the mechanisms and nursing considerations for antiemetics
- Explain the appropriate use of laxatives and antidiarrheals
- Recognize the adverse effects of GI medications requiring intervention
- Apply safety principles for medications used in inflammatory bowel disease
- Describe the treatment of H. pylori infection
- Educate patients about proper use of GI medications

6.2 Overview of GI Pharmacology

The gastrointestinal system is responsible for digestion, absorption, and elimination. GI medications target acid secretion, motility, nausea, and inflammation. Understanding the mechanisms helps nurses anticipate effects and educate patients effectively.

6.3 Acid-Reducing Medications

Proton Pump Inhibitors (PPIs)

Drugs: Omeprazole (Prilosec), esomeprazole (Nexium), lansoprazole (Prevacid), pantoprazole (Protonix), rabeprazole (Aciphex)

Memory Tip: End in "-prazole"

Mechanism: Irreversibly inhibit the proton pump (H^+/K^+ ATPase) in parietal cells → most potent acid suppression

Uses: GERD, peptic ulcer disease, H. pylori eradication, Zollinger-Ellison syndrome, stress ulcer prophylaxis

Administration: Take 30-60 minutes BEFORE meals (usually before breakfast). Do not crush enteric-coated tablets.

Adverse Effects:

- Short-term: Headache, diarrhea, nausea, abdominal pain
- Long-term concerns:
- Increased fracture risk (decreased calcium absorption)
- Hypomagnesemia (monitor magnesium with long-term use)
- Vitamin B12 deficiency
- C. difficile infection risk
- Possible increased risk of kidney disease

Drug Interactions: Decrease absorption of drugs requiring acid (iron, calcium, ketoconazole). Omeprazole inhibits CYP2C19—interacts with clopidogrel.

Clinical Pearl: PPIs are often overprescribed. Review need periodically—many patients can step down to H2 blockers or as-needed use.

Histamine-2 Receptor Antagonists (H2 Blockers)

Drugs: Famotidine (Pepcid), ranitidine (Zantac—withdrawn in many countries), cimetidine (Tagamet), nizatidine (Axid)

Memory Tip: End in "-tidine"

Mechanism: Block H2 receptors on parietal cells → decreased acid secretion

Uses: GERD (mild), peptic ulcer disease, stress ulcer prophylaxis

Less potent than PPIs but fewer long-term concerns

Cimetidine Considerations: Potent CYP450 inhibitor (many drug interactions), can cause gynecomastia and confusion in elderly. Famotidine preferred.

Clinical Pearl: H2 blockers can be taken at bedtime to suppress nocturnal acid secretion.

Antacids

Drugs: Aluminum hydroxide, magnesium hydroxide (Milk of Magnesia), calcium carbonate (Tums), sodium bicarbonate

Mechanism: Neutralize existing stomach acid (do not reduce acid production)

Uses: Quick relief of heartburn and indigestion

Adverse Effects:

- Aluminum-based: Constipation
- Magnesium-based: Diarrhea
- Calcium-based: Constipation, rebound acid secretion, milk-alkali syndrome (with excess use)

- Sodium bicarbonate: Sodium load (avoid in heart failure, hypertension)

Drug Interactions: Decrease absorption of many medications. Separate from other drugs by 2 hours.

Clinical Pearl: "Aluminum = constipAtion, Magnesium = Moves things along"

Mucosal Protectants

Sucralfate (Carafate):

- Forms a protective barrier over ulcers
- Take on empty stomach, 1 hour before meals
- Separate from other medications by 2 hours
- May cause constipation

Misoprostol (Cytotec):

- Prostaglandin analog—protects gastric mucosa
- Used to prevent NSAID-induced ulcers
- CONTRAINDICATED in pregnancy (causes uterine contractions, abortion)
- BLACK BOX WARNING for pregnancy

6.4 H. pylori Treatment

Triple Therapy: PPI + clarithromycin + amoxicillin (or metronidazole) for 14 days

Quadruple Therapy: PPI + bismuth subsalicylate + metronidazole + tetracycline

Nursing Considerations:

- Complete full course of therapy
- Bismuth causes black stools (expected, not blood)
- Avoid alcohol with metronidazole (disulfiram-like reaction)
- Confirm eradication with follow-up testing

6.5 Antiemetics

Serotonin (5-HT3) Antagonists

Drugs: Ondansetron (Zofran), granisetron (Kytril), palonosetron (Aloxi)

Memory Tip: End in "-setron"

Mechanism: Block serotonin receptors in the chemoreceptor trigger zone and GI tract

Uses: Chemotherapy-induced nausea/vomiting (CINV), postoperative nausea, radiation-induced nausea

Adverse Effects: Headache, constipation, QT prolongation (monitor ECG in high-risk patients)

Clinical Pearl: Ondansetron is often first-line for nausea/vomiting due to effectiveness and safety profile.

Dopamine Antagonists

Drugs: Metoclopramide (Reglan), prochlorperazine (Compazine), promethazine (Phenergan)

Mechanism: Block dopamine receptors in the CTZ; metoclopramide also increases GI motility

Uses: Nausea/vomiting, gastroparesis (metoclopramide), migraine-associated nausea

Adverse Effects:

- Extrapyramidal symptoms (EPS)—dystonia, akathisia, parkinsonism
- Tardive dyskinesia (with long-term metoclopramide)—BLACK BOX WARNING
- Sedation

Metoclopramide: Limit use to 12 weeks maximum due to tardive dyskinesia risk.

Promethazine: Tissue necrosis with IV extravasation—give deep IM or dilute IV slowly. BLACK BOX for children < 2 years.

Anticholinergic/Antihistamine Antiemetics

Drugs: Scopolamine (Transderm Scop patch), meclizine (Antivert), dimenhydrinate (Dramamine)

Uses: Motion sickness, vertigo

Adverse Effects: Dry mouth, drowsiness, urinary retention, blurred vision (anticholinergic effects)

Scopolamine Patch: Apply behind ear 4 hours before travel. Wash hands after handling (can dilate pupils if touched).

Neurokinin-1 (NK1) Antagonists

Drugs: Aprepitant (Emend), fosaprepitant, rolapitant

Uses: Prevention of CINV (used with 5-HT3 antagonist and dexamethasone for highly emetogenic chemo)

Drug Interactions: CYP3A4 substrate and inhibitor—many interactions including with warfarin, oral contraceptives

Cannabinoids

Drugs: Dronabinol (Marinol), nabilone (Cesamet)

Uses: CINV refractory to other treatments, appetite stimulation in AIDS wasting

Adverse Effects: Euphoria, dizziness, drowsiness, paranoia. Controlled substance.

6.6 Laxatives

Bulk-Forming Laxatives

Drugs: Psyllium (Metamucil), methylcellulose (Citrucel)

Mechanism: Absorb water → increase stool bulk → stimulate peristalsis

Uses: Chronic constipation, IBS

CRITICAL: Must take with FULL glass of water (8 oz) to prevent obstruction. Onset: 12-72 hours.

Osmotic Laxatives

Drugs: Polyethylene glycol (MiraLAX), lactulose, magnesium hydroxide (Milk of Magnesia), magnesium citrate

Mechanism: Draw water into intestinal lumen → soften stool

Uses: Constipation, bowel prep (PEG-electrolyte solutions like GoLYTELY)

Lactulose: Also used for hepatic encephalopathy (promotes ammonia excretion)

Caution: Magnesium-containing laxatives—avoid in renal impairment (magnesium accumulation)

Stimulant Laxatives

Drugs: Bisacodyl (Dulcolax), senna (Senokot)

Mechanism: Stimulate intestinal nerve plexus → increased motility and secretion

Uses: Short-term constipation, bowel prep, opioid-induced constipation

Caution: Not for long-term use (can cause dependence, electrolyte imbalances). Onset: 6-12 hours (oral).

Stool Softeners

Drug: Docusate sodium (Colace)

Mechanism: Surfactant that allows water and fat to penetrate stool

Uses: Prevention of constipation in patients who should not strain (cardiac, post-surgical)

Note: Prevents hard stools but does not treat existing constipation effectively

Opioid-Induced Constipation (OIC) Medications

Drugs: Methylnaltrexone (Relistor), naloxegol (Movantik), naldemedine (Symproic)

Mechanism: Peripheral opioid receptor antagonists—block opioid effects in GI tract without affecting analgesia

Uses: OIC when other laxatives have failed

6.7 Antidiarrheals

Opioid Agonists

Drugs: Loperamide (Imodium), diphenoxylate/atropine (Lomotil)

Mechanism: Activate opioid receptors in GI tract → decrease motility

Uses: Acute noninfectious diarrhea, traveler's diarrhea

CONTRAINDICATED: Infectious diarrhea with fever or bloody stools (traps bacteria), C. difficile colitis

Loperamide: Does not cross blood-brain barrier at normal doses—no CNS effects. OTC.

Diphenoxylate/Atropine: Atropine added to discourage abuse. Controlled substance.

Bismuth Subsalicylate

Drug: Pepto-Bismol

Uses: Diarrhea, upset stomach, H. pylori regimens

Adverse Effects: Black tongue and stools (harmless), tinnitus (salicylate toxicity if excessive)

Caution: Contains salicylate—avoid with aspirin allergy, children with viral illness (Reye syndrome)

6.8 Inflammatory Bowel Disease Medications

Aminosalicylates (5-ASA)

Drugs: Mesalamine (Asacol, Pentasa, Lialda), sulfasalazine (Azulfidine)

Mechanism: Local anti-inflammatory effect in GI tract

Uses: Ulcerative colitis, mild Crohn's disease

Sulfasalazine: Also used for rheumatoid arthritis. Can cause orange-yellow urine. Sulfa allergy caution.

Nursing Considerations: Adequate hydration, monitor renal function, take with food

Corticosteroids

Drugs: Prednisone, budesonide (Entocort—local action, less systemic effects)

Uses: Acute flares of IBD

Note: Not for maintenance—use immunomodulators or biologics for long-term control

Immunomodulators

Drugs: Azathioprine (Imuran), 6-mercaptopurine, methotrexate

Uses: Maintenance of remission in IBD

Adverse Effects: Bone marrow suppression (monitor CBC), hepatotoxicity, increased infection risk

TPMT Testing: Check before starting azathioprine/6-MP—deficiency increases toxicity risk

Biologic Therapies

TNF-alpha Inhibitors: Infliximab (Remicade), adalimumab (Humira)

Integrin Inhibitors: Vedolizumab (Entyvio)—gut-selective

IL-12/23 Inhibitors: Ustekinumab (Stelara)

BLACK BOX WARNINGS: Serious infections (TB, opportunistic), malignancy (lymphoma). Screen for TB before starting.

6.9 Medications for IBS

IBS-C (Constipation):

- Lubiprostone (Amitiza): Chloride channel activator—increases intestinal fluid
- Linaclotide (Linzess): Guanylate cyclase agonist—increases fluid secretion

IBS-D (Diarrhea):

- Alosetron (Lotronex): 5-HT3 antagonist—slows motility. REMS program due to ischemic colitis risk. Only for severe IBS-D in women.
- Rifaximin (Xifaxan): Non-absorbed antibiotic for IBS-D

Antispasmodics: Dicyclomine (Bentyl), hyoscyamine—anticholinergics for cramping

6.10 Pancreatic Enzyme Replacement

Drug: Pancrelipase (Creon, Zenpep, Pancreaze)

Uses: Pancreatic insufficiency (chronic pancreatitis, cystic fibrosis, post-pancreatectomy)

Administration:

- Take with meals and snacks
- Do not crush or chew enteric-coated capsules

- Can open capsule and sprinkle on acidic food (applesauce)

Adverse Effects: GI upset, hyperuricemia with high doses. Fibrosing colonopathy with very high doses (rare).

6.11 Chapter Summary

- PPIs: Most potent acid suppression. Take before meals. Long-term risks include fractures, hypomagnesemia, C. diff.
- H2 Blockers: Less potent than PPIs. Famotidine preferred (fewer interactions than cimetidine).
- Ondansetron: First-line antiemetic. Watch QT prolongation.
- Metoclopramide: Limit to 12 weeks—tardive dyskinesia risk (BLACK BOX).
- Laxatives: Bulk-forming need full glass of water. Stimulants not for long-term use.
- Loperamide: Do NOT use in infectious or bloody diarrhea.
- IBD Biologics: Screen for TB before starting. BLACK BOX for infections and malignancy.

6.12 Practice Questions

Directions: Select the best answer for each question.

1. A patient taking omeprazole should be instructed to take the medication:

A. At bedtime with a snack
B. 30-60 minutes before breakfast
C. With meals three times daily
D. Only when experiencing heartburn

2. A patient on long-term PPI therapy should be monitored for:

A. Hyperkalemia
B. Hypomagnesemia
C. Hypercalcemia
D. Hypernatremia

3. Which antiemetic is most appropriate for chemotherapy-induced nausea?

A. Scopolamine
B. Meclizine
C. Ondansetron
D. Diphenhydramine

4. A patient prescribed metoclopramide for gastroparesis should be taught:

A. This medication may be used indefinitely

B. Limit use to 12 weeks due to movement disorder risk

C. Take the medication at bedtime only

D. Expect immediate relief of symptoms

5. A patient taking psyllium (Metamucil) for constipation must:

A. Limit fluid intake to prevent bloating

B. Take it with a full glass of water

C. Take it on an empty stomach at bedtime

D. Crush the tablets before swallowing

6. Which laxative is most appropriate for a patient with opioid-induced constipation?

A. Docusate sodium (Colace) alone

B. Psyllium (Metamucil)

C. Senna (Senokot)

D. Aluminum hydroxide

7. A patient with acute diarrhea and fever should NOT receive:

A. Oral rehydration therapy

B. Loperamide (Imodium)

C. Probiotics

D. Bland diet

8. Sucralfate should be administered:

A. With meals for best effect

B. One hour before meals on an empty stomach

C. At bedtime with antacids

D. Mixed with milk or juice

9. A patient taking bismuth subsalicylate (Pepto-Bismol) should be taught that:

A. Black stools indicate GI bleeding

B. Black stools are an expected effect

C. The medication should be taken with aspirin

D. Children with flu can safely take this

10. Which medication requires TB screening before initiation?

A. Mesalamine

B. Sulfasalazine

C. Infliximab

D. Budesonide

11. A nurse should question an order for misoprostol in a patient who:

A. Has NSAID-induced ulcer

B. Is pregnant

C. Has GERD

D. Is male

12. The nurse teaches a patient using a scopolamine patch to:

A. Apply it to the forearm

B. Apply it behind the ear and wash hands after

C. Replace it daily

D. Expect it to work immediately

13. A patient on lactulose for hepatic encephalopathy should expect:

A. Two to three soft stools daily

B. Complete relief from confusion immediately

C. Dark, tarry stools

D. No change in bowel habits

14. Which statement indicates a patient understands H. pylori treatment?

A. I only need to take antibiotics when I have symptoms

B. I must complete the full course of all medications

C. I can stop the PPI once I feel better

D. Bismuth will make my stools red

15. A patient taking sulfasalazine for ulcerative colitis should:

A. Expect orange-yellow discoloration of urine

B. Avoid all sun exposure

C. Limit fluid intake

D. Stop the medication if diarrhea occurs

16. Promethazine IV administration requires:

A. Rapid IV push for best effect

B. Dilution and slow administration due to tissue damage risk

C. Administration only through central line

D. Mixing with other medications

17. A patient with IBS-C is prescribed linaclotide. The nurse teaches:

A. Take with a high-fat meal

B. Take on an empty stomach 30 minutes before breakfast

C. Expect immediate constipation relief

D. Crush tablets for easier swallowing

18. Which finding would concern the nurse in a patient on long-term PPI therapy?

A. Relief of heartburn symptoms

B. Occasional headache

C. Muscle cramps and tremors

D. Mild diarrhea

19. Pancrelipase (Creon) should be administered:

A. On an empty stomach

B. With meals and snacks

C. Once daily at bedtime

D. Only when steatorrhea occurs

20. A patient taking aluminum-containing antacids is most likely to experience:

A. Diarrhea

B. Constipation

C. Hyperkalemia

D. Fluid retention

CHAPTER 7

Anti-Infective Medications

7.1 Learning Objectives

By the end of this chapter, you will be able to:

- Differentiate between bactericidal and bacteriostatic antibiotics
- Identify the major antibiotic drug classes and their mechanisms
- Explain the nursing considerations for aminoglycosides and vancomycin
- Recognize adverse effects of anti-infectives requiring intervention
- Apply principles of antibiotic stewardship
- Describe the treatment of common fungal, viral, and parasitic infections
- Educate patients about proper antibiotic use and completion of therapy

7.2 Overview of Anti-Infective Pharmacology

Anti-infective medications target bacteria, viruses, fungi, and parasites. Understanding the mechanisms helps nurses anticipate effects, monitor for toxicity, and educate patients about proper use. Antibiotic stewardship—using antibiotics appropriately—is critical to prevent resistance.

Bactericidal: Kill bacteria (penicillins, cephalosporins, aminoglycosides, fluoroquinolones, vancomycin)

Bacteriostatic: Inhibit bacterial growth (tetracyclines, macrolides, sulfonamides)—immune system must eliminate bacteria

7.3 Penicillins

Drugs: Penicillin G/V, amoxicillin, ampicillin, piperacillin-tazobactam (Zosyn)

Mechanism: Inhibit bacterial cell wall synthesis → bactericidal

Uses: Streptococcal infections, syphilis, otitis media, respiratory infections

Adverse Effects:

- Allergic reactions (most common antibiotic allergy)—rash to anaphylaxis
- GI upset, diarrhea

- Superinfection (C. difficile, yeast)

Cross-Reactivity: ~10% cross-reactivity with cephalosporins (historically cited; actual risk may be lower, especially with newer cephalosporins)

Nursing Considerations:

- Always assess allergy history before administration
- Monitor for allergic reactions, especially with first dose
- Take amoxicillin without regard to food; penicillin V on empty stomach

Clinical Pearl: Amoxicillin-clavulanate (Augmentin) adds beta-lactamase inhibitor to extend coverage to resistant organisms.

7.4 Cephalosporins

Generations:

- 1st Generation (cefazolin, cephalexin): Gram-positive coverage, surgical prophylaxis
- 2nd Generation (cefuroxime, cefoxitin): Expanded gram-negative
- 3rd Generation (ceftriaxone, cefotaxime): Broader gram-negative, CNS penetration
- 4th Generation (cefepime): Broad spectrum including Pseudomonas
- 5th Generation (ceftaroline): MRSA coverage

Memory Tip: "Generations go up, gram-negative coverage goes up"

Mechanism: Inhibit cell wall synthesis (like penicillins)

Adverse Effects: Allergic reactions, GI upset, superinfection, bleeding (cefotetan, cefoperazone)

Nursing Considerations:

- Cross-reactivity with penicillin allergy—assess severity of prior reaction
- Ceftriaxone: Do NOT mix with calcium-containing solutions (precipitation)
- Some cephalosporins interact with alcohol (disulfiram-like reaction)

7.5 Fluoroquinolones

Drugs: Ciprofloxacin (Cipro), levofloxacin (Levaquin), moxifloxacin (Avelox)

Memory Tip: End in "-floxacin"

Mechanism: Inhibit DNA gyrase and topoisomerase IV → bactericidal

Uses: UTIs, respiratory infections, GI infections, anthrax

BLACK BOX WARNINGS:

- Tendinitis and tendon rupture (especially Achilles)—risk increased in elderly, corticosteroid use, kidney/heart/lung transplant
- Peripheral neuropathy (may be irreversible)
- CNS effects (seizures, confusion, psychosis)
- Exacerbation of myasthenia gravis
- Aortic aneurysm/dissection

Other Adverse Effects: QT prolongation, photosensitivity, C. difficile colitis

Drug Interactions: Antacids, calcium, iron, zinc decrease absorption—separate by 2 hours. Increases theophylline and warfarin levels.

Clinical Pearl: Reserve fluoroquinolones for when other options are not suitable due to serious adverse effects.

7.6 Aminoglycosides

Drugs: Gentamicin, tobramycin, amikacin, streptomycin

Memory Tip: End in "-mycin" (but not all -mycins are aminoglycosides)

Mechanism: Inhibit protein synthesis (30S ribosome) → bactericidal

Uses: Serious gram-negative infections, often with other antibiotics for synergy

Administration: IV or IM (not absorbed orally). Often once-daily dosing.

NARROW THERAPEUTIC INDEX: Requires peak and trough monitoring

Major Toxicities:

- NEPHROTOXICITY: Monitor BUN, creatinine, urine output. Usually reversible.
- OTOTOXICITY: Hearing loss (cochlear) and vestibular damage. May be irreversible. Report tinnitus, hearing changes, vertigo.

Risk Factors for Toxicity: Prolonged therapy, high doses, dehydration, concurrent nephrotoxic drugs (vancomycin, NSAIDs, amphotericin B)

Nursing Considerations:

- Monitor drug levels (peak and trough)
- Monitor renal function (creatinine) daily
- Ensure adequate hydration
- Assess hearing baseline and during therapy

Clinical Pearl: "Aminoglycosides attack the ears and kidneys"—ototoxicity and nephrotoxicity are the major concerns.

7.7 Vancomycin

Mechanism: Inhibits cell wall synthesis → bactericidal

Uses: MRSA, serious gram-positive infections, C. difficile colitis (oral form only)

Administration: IV for systemic infections; oral for C. difficile (not absorbed—stays in GI tract)

NARROW THERAPEUTIC INDEX: Trough monitoring required (goal varies by indication)

Adverse Effects:

- RED MAN SYNDROME: Flushing, pruritus, hypotension from rapid infusion. NOT a true allergy. Prevent by infusing over ≥60 minutes.
- NEPHROTOXICITY: Monitor creatinine, especially with concurrent aminoglycosides
- OTOTOXICITY: Less common than aminoglycosides

Nursing Considerations:

- Infuse over at least 60 minutes (longer for higher doses)
- Monitor trough levels before 4th or 5th dose
- Monitor renal function
- If Red Man Syndrome occurs: stop infusion, give antihistamine, restart slowly

Clinical Pearl: Red Man Syndrome is rate-related, not a true allergy. Slow the infusion rate.

7.8 Macrolides

Drugs: Azithromycin (Zithromax, Z-pack), clarithromycin (Biaxin), erythromycin

Mechanism: Inhibit protein synthesis (50S ribosome) → bacteriostatic

Uses: Respiratory infections, atypical pneumonia (Mycoplasma, Legionella), H. pylori, STIs

Adverse Effects:

- GI upset (especially erythromycin)—take with food
- QT prolongation (all macrolides)—avoid in patients with cardiac risk
- Hepatotoxicity

Drug Interactions: Erythromycin and clarithromycin are strong CYP3A4 inhibitors—many interactions (statins, warfarin, theophylline). Azithromycin has fewer interactions.

Clinical Pearl: Azithromycin is preferred due to once-daily dosing, fewer GI effects, and fewer drug interactions.

7.9 Tetracyclines

Drugs: Doxycycline, tetracycline, minocycline

Mechanism: Inhibit protein synthesis (30S ribosome) → bacteriostatic

Uses: Acne, Lyme disease, Rocky Mountain spotted fever, chlamydia, MRSA (doxycycline)

Adverse Effects:

- Photosensitivity (severe sunburn)—use sunscreen, protective clothing
- GI upset—take with food (except tetracycline)
- Esophageal irritation—take with full glass of water, remain upright
- Tooth discoloration and bone growth inhibition in children

CONTRAINDICATED: Pregnancy and children < 8 years (permanent tooth staining, bone effects)

Drug Interactions: Dairy, antacids, iron, calcium decrease absorption—separate by 2 hours.

Clinical Pearl: Doxycycline can be taken with food (unlike older tetracyclines) and is less affected by dairy.

7.10 Sulfonamides and Trimethoprim

Drug: Sulfamethoxazole-trimethoprim (Bactrim, Septra) = TMP-SMX

Mechanism: Inhibit folic acid synthesis → bacteriostatic (bactericidal in combination)

Uses: UTIs, MRSA skin infections, PCP pneumonia prophylaxis, travelers' diarrhea

Adverse Effects:

- SULFA ALLERGY: Rash, Stevens-Johnson syndrome, anaphylaxis—assess allergy history
- Bone marrow suppression (monitor CBC)
- Hyperkalemia
- Photosensitivity
- Crystalluria—encourage fluids

Contraindications: Sulfa allergy, pregnancy (near term), infants < 2 months, G6PD deficiency

Drug Interactions: Increases warfarin effect, increases methotrexate toxicity

7.11 Other Antibacterials

Metronidazole (Flagyl)

Uses: Anaerobic infections, C. difficile, trichomoniasis, bacterial vaginosis, H. pylori

Adverse Effects: Metallic taste, GI upset, dark urine

CRITICAL: AVOID ALCOHOL—disulfiram-like reaction (severe nausea, vomiting, flushing). Avoid during and 3 days after therapy.

Neurotoxicity: Peripheral neuropathy with prolonged use

Clindamycin (Cleocin)

Uses: Anaerobic infections, MRSA skin infections, bone infections

BLACK BOX WARNING: High risk of C. difficile-associated diarrhea (CDAD). Monitor for diarrhea.

Nitrofurantoin (Macrobid)

Uses: UTIs only (concentrates in urine, not effective systemically)

Adverse Effects: GI upset (take with food), pulmonary toxicity (chronic use)

Contraindications: CrCl < 30 mL/min (ineffective and increased toxicity)

Linezolid (Zyvox)

Uses: MRSA, VRE (vancomycin-resistant enterococcus)

Adverse Effects: Bone marrow suppression (monitor CBC weekly), serotonin syndrome with SSRIs/MAOIs, peripheral neuropathy

Note: Weak MAOI—avoid tyramine-rich foods

7.12 Antifungals

Azole Antifungals

Drugs: Fluconazole (Diflucan), itraconazole, voriconazole, ketoconazole

Memory Tip: End in "-azole"

Uses: Candidiasis, cryptococcosis, various fungal infections

Adverse Effects: Hepatotoxicity (monitor LFTs), QT prolongation, GI upset

Drug Interactions: Strong CYP450 inhibitors—MANY interactions. Check before prescribing.

Fluconazole: Most commonly used; single dose for vaginal candidiasis

Amphotericin B

Uses: Severe systemic fungal infections (aspergillosis, cryptococcal meningitis)

"Amphoterrible": Significant toxicity:

- NEPHROTOXICITY (major concern)—monitor BUN, creatinine, electrolytes
- Infusion reactions (fever, chills, rigors)—premedicate with diphenhydramine, acetaminophen, meperidine
- Hypokalemia, hypomagnesemia

Lipid Formulations: Less nephrotoxic but expensive

Echinocandins

Drugs: Caspofungin, micafungin, anidulafungin

Uses: Invasive candidiasis, aspergillosis

Advantages: Fewer drug interactions, less nephrotoxicity than amphotericin B

7.13 Antivirals

Antivirals for Herpes/Varicella

Drugs: Acyclovir (Zovirax), valacyclovir (Valtrex), famciclovir (Famvir)

Uses: HSV, VZV (shingles), CMV prophylaxis

Adverse Effects: Nephrotoxicity (ensure adequate hydration), neurotoxicity at high doses

Nursing Considerations: Encourage fluids, start treatment early for best results

Antivirals for Influenza

Drugs: Oseltamivir (Tamiflu), zanamivir (Relenza), baloxavir (Xofluza)

Uses: Influenza A and B treatment and prophylaxis

Timing: Most effective if started within 48 hours of symptom onset

Antiretrovirals for HIV

Drug Classes: NRTIs, NNRTIs, protease inhibitors, integrase inhibitors, entry inhibitors

Principles:

- Combination therapy (ART) required—never monotherapy
- Adherence critical to prevent resistance

- Many drug interactions (especially protease inhibitors)
- Monitor viral load and CD4 count

7.14 Antitubercular Drugs

First-Line Drugs: RIPE = Rifampin, Isoniazid (INH), Pyrazinamide, Ethambutol

Treatment Duration: Minimum 6 months; longer for extrapulmonary or resistant TB

Drug-Specific Concerns:

- Rifampin: Orange-red body fluids (normal), potent CYP450 inducer (many interactions)
- Isoniazid: Peripheral neuropathy (give vitamin B6/pyridoxine), hepatotoxicity
- Pyrazinamide: Hepatotoxicity, hyperuricemia
- Ethambutol: Optic neuritis—monitor visual acuity and color discrimination

Nursing Considerations:

- Directly observed therapy (DOT) often used to ensure adherence
- Monitor LFTs for all drugs
- Completion of full course essential to prevent resistance

7.15 Antibiotic Stewardship

Key principles for nurses:

- Obtain cultures before starting antibiotics when possible
- Use narrow-spectrum when appropriate
- Ensure correct dose, route, and duration
- Reassess antibiotic therapy at 48-72 hours
- Complete full course of therapy
- Educate patients: antibiotics don't treat viruses
- Monitor for C. difficile, especially with broad-spectrum antibiotics

7.16 Chapter Summary

- Penicillin allergy: Most common antibiotic allergy. Assess carefully before administration.
- Fluoroquinolones: BLACK BOX for tendon rupture, neuropathy, CNS effects. Reserve for appropriate indications.
- Aminoglycosides: Monitor peak/trough levels. Nephrotoxicity and ototoxicity are major concerns.

- Vancomycin: Infuse slowly to prevent Red Man Syndrome. Monitor trough levels and renal function.
- Tetracyclines: Photosensitivity. Avoid in pregnancy and children < 8 years.
- Metronidazole: NO ALCOHOL—disulfiram-like reaction.
- Antifungals: Azoles inhibit CYP450 (many interactions). Amphotericin B is nephrotoxic.

7.17 Practice Questions

Directions: Select the best answer for each question.

1. A patient receiving vancomycin develops flushing, pruritus, and hypotension during infusion. The nurse should:

A. Stop the infusion and never give vancomycin again

B. Stop the infusion, give antihistamine, and restart at slower rate

C. Continue the infusion as this is expected

D. Increase the infusion rate to finish quickly

2. A patient on gentamicin therapy should be monitored for:

A. Hepatotoxicity and jaundice

B. Nephrotoxicity and ototoxicity

C. Cardiac arrhythmias

D. Bone marrow suppression

3. Which instruction is most important for a patient taking ciprofloxacin?

A. Take with dairy products for better absorption

B. Report any tendon pain immediately

C. Expect orange discoloration of urine

D. Take the medication at bedtime only

4. A patient taking metronidazole should be taught to avoid:

A. Dairy products

B. Alcohol

C. Citrus fruits

D. Caffeine

5. Which antibiotic is contraindicated in children under 8 years?

A. Amoxicillin

B. Azithromycin

C. Doxycycline

D. Cephalexin

6. A patient asks why they must complete the full course of antibiotics. The nurse explains:

A. Stopping early can lead to antibiotic resistance

B. The medication needs time to fully absorb

C. Symptoms always return if stopped early

D. It is required by law to complete all prescriptions

7. The nurse should question an order for fluoroquinolone in a patient taking:

A. Metformin

B. Lisinopril

C. Corticosteroids

D. Metoprolol

8. A patient on rifampin for tuberculosis should be taught to expect:

A. Blue discoloration of skin

B. Orange-red discoloration of body fluids

C. Permanent hair loss

D. Increased appetite

9. Which finding indicates a patient is experiencing amphotericin B toxicity?

A. Elevated liver enzymes

B. Elevated serum creatinine

C. Decreased white blood cell count

D. Elevated blood glucose

10. Before administering the first dose of penicillin, the nurse should:

A. Check for allergies to penicillin and cephalosporins

B. Administer a test dose intradermally

C. Give prophylactic diphenhydramine

D. Verify the patient has eaten recently

11. A patient on isoniazid for TB prophylaxis should also receive:

A. Vitamin B12

B. Vitamin B6 (pyridoxine)

C. Vitamin C

D. Folic acid

12. A patient taking sulfamethoxazole-trimethoprim should:

A. Restrict fluid intake

B. Increase fluid intake to prevent crystalluria

C. Avoid all protein in diet

D. Take the medication with antacids

13. Which patient statement indicates understanding of azithromycin therapy?

A. I will take this medication with antacids

B. I will complete all 5 days of the Z-pack

C. I can stop when I feel better

D. I should take this on an empty stomach only

14. A nurse should hold vancomycin and notify the provider if the trough level is:

A. 8 mcg/mL

B. 12 mcg/mL

C. 15 mcg/mL

D. 25 mcg/mL

15. Which antifungal requires monitoring for visual changes?

A. Fluconazole

B. Amphotericin B

C. Voriconazole

D. Caspofungin

16. A patient with a documented severe penicillin allergy (anaphylaxis) should avoid:

A. Azithromycin

B. Vancomycin

C. Ceftriaxone

D. Ciprofloxacin

17. The priority nursing intervention for a patient starting aminoglycoside therapy is:

A. Ensuring adequate oral intake

B. Assessing baseline hearing and renal function

C. Teaching about photosensitivity

D. Monitoring liver function tests

18. A patient taking fluconazole should be monitored for:

A. Nephrotoxicity

B. Hepatotoxicity

C. Ototoxicity

D. Cardiotoxicity

19. Which statement about C. difficile infection is correct?

A. It is treated with IV vancomycin

B. Oral vancomycin or fidaxomicin is the treatment

C. It only occurs with penicillin use

D. Antidiarrheal medications speed recovery

20. A patient on acyclovir for shingles should be taught to:

A. Limit fluid intake to prevent edema

B. Drink plenty of fluids to protect kidneys

C. Apply the oral medication to the lesions

D. Expect complete resolution within 24 hours

CHAPTER 8

Fluids, Electrolytes, and Renal Medications

8.1 Learning Objectives

By the end of this chapter, you will be able to:

- Differentiate between crystalloid and colloid IV solutions
- Identify the appropriate IV fluid for various clinical situations
- Explain the mechanisms and nursing considerations for diuretics
- Recognize signs and symptoms of electrolyte imbalances
- Apply safety principles for potassium administration
- Describe medications used in chronic kidney disease
- Educate patients about fluid and electrolyte management

8.2 Overview of Fluid and Electrolyte Pharmacology

Maintaining fluid and electrolyte balance is essential for cellular function, cardiac rhythm, neuromuscular activity, and organ perfusion. Nurses must understand IV fluid therapy, electrolyte replacement, and diuretics to safely manage patients with imbalances.

8.3 Intravenous Fluids

Crystalloids

Definition: Solutions containing water, electrolytes, and sometimes glucose. Freely cross capillary membranes.

Isotonic Solutions (same osmolarity as blood ~275-295 mOsm/L):

- 0.9% Normal Saline (NS): 154 mEq Na+/Cl-. Expands intravascular volume. Use for hypovolemia, blood transfusions, Na+ replacement.
- Lactated Ringer's (LR): Contains Na+, K+, Ca++, lactate. Preferred for fluid resuscitation, surgery. Avoid in liver failure (can't metabolize lactate).
- D5W: Isotonic in bag but becomes hypotonic once dextrose metabolized. Provides free water and calories. Not for resuscitation.

Hypotonic Solutions (< 275 mOsm/L):

- 0.45% NS (half-normal saline): Provides free water. Use for hypernatremia, cellular dehydration.
- CAUTION: Can cause cellular swelling. Avoid in increased ICP, third-spacing.

Hypertonic Solutions (> 295 mOsm/L):

- 3% Saline: For severe symptomatic hyponatremia. Give via central line, monitor closely.
- D10W, D50W: For hypoglycemia.
- CAUTION: Can cause cellular shrinkage, fluid shifts. Monitor for fluid overload.

Clinical Pearl: "Isotonic stays in vessels, hypotonic goes into cells, hypertonic pulls fluid from cells."

Colloids

Definition: Solutions containing large molecules that stay in intravascular space longer.

- Albumin (5%, 25%): Blood product. Expands plasma volume. Use for hypovolemia, burns, liver failure.
- Dextran: Synthetic. Plasma expander. Can interfere with blood typing.
- Hetastarch: Synthetic. Fluid resuscitation. Risk of coagulopathy, renal injury.

Advantages: Remain in vascular space longer than crystalloids.

Disadvantages: More expensive, risk of allergic reactions, some affect coagulation.

8.4 Diuretics

Loop Diuretics

Drugs: Furosemide (Lasix), bumetanide (Bumex), torsemide (Demadex)

Mechanism: Block Na+/K+/2Cl- transporter in loop of Henle → potent diuresis

Uses: Heart failure, pulmonary edema, edema, hypertension, acute kidney injury

"Ceiling is the roof": Most potent diuretics

Adverse Effects:

- HYPOKALEMIA (major concern)—monitor K+, may need supplements
- Hyponatremia, hypocalcemia, hypomagnesemia
- Hypotension, dehydration
- Ototoxicity (especially with rapid IV administration or concurrent aminoglycosides)
- Hyperglycemia, hyperuricemia (gout)

Nursing Considerations:

- Monitor I&O, daily weights, electrolytes

- Give in morning to prevent nocturia
- IV push: Give slowly over 1-2 minutes to prevent ototoxicity
- Monitor for signs of dehydration and electrolyte imbalances

Clinical Pearl: Furosemide and digoxin together: Low K+ increases digoxin toxicity. Always monitor potassium.

Thiazide Diuretics

Drugs: Hydrochlorothiazide (HCTZ), chlorthalidone, metolazone

Mechanism: Block Na+/Cl- transporter in distal tubule → moderate diuresis

Uses: Hypertension (first-line), mild edema, nephrogenic diabetes insipidus, kidney stones

Adverse Effects:

- HYPOKALEMIA
- Hypercalcemia (opposite of loops)—good for osteoporosis
- Hyperglycemia, hyperuricemia
- Hyponatremia (especially in elderly)
- Photosensitivity

Sulfa Allergy: Thiazides are sulfonamide derivatives—use caution in sulfa allergy.

Clinical Pearl: Metolazone can be added to loop diuretics for synergistic effect in resistant edema.

Potassium-Sparing Diuretics

Drugs:

- Spironolactone (Aldactone), eplerenone (Inspra): Aldosterone antagonists
- Triamterene, amiloride: Direct action on collecting duct

Mechanism: Block sodium reabsorption while retaining potassium in collecting duct

Uses: Heart failure, hypertension, cirrhotic ascites, hypokalemia prevention

Adverse Effects:

- HYPERKALEMIA (major concern)—monitor K+, avoid K+ supplements and salt substitutes
- Spironolactone: Gynecomastia, menstrual irregularities (antiandrogen effects)

Contraindications: Hyperkalemia, severe renal impairment, concurrent ACE inhibitors/ARBs (additive hyperkalemia risk)

Clinical Pearl: Spironolactone improves survival in heart failure (blocks harmful aldosterone effects).

Osmotic Diuretics

Drug: Mannitol (Osmitrol)

Mechanism: Osmotically pulls water into renal tubules → increased urine output

Uses: Increased intracranial pressure, acute glaucoma, prevention of acute renal failure

Administration: IV only. Use filter needle (crystallizes). Warm if crystals present.

Adverse Effects: Fluid and electrolyte imbalances, pulmonary edema (initial fluid shift into vessels)

CONTRAINDICATED: Heart failure, pulmonary edema, anuria (need functioning kidneys)

Carbonic Anhydrase Inhibitors

Drug: Acetazolamide (Diamox)

Uses: Glaucoma, altitude sickness, metabolic alkalosis

Adverse Effects: Metabolic acidosis, hypokalemia, paresthesias

Sulfa derivative: Caution in sulfa allergy

8.5 Electrolyte Replacement

Potassium

Normal Range: 3.5-5.0 mEq/L

Hypokalemia Signs: Muscle weakness, leg cramps, fatigue, constipation, U waves on ECG, cardiac arrhythmias

Replacement:

- Oral: KCl tablets or liquid. Take with food and full glass of water (GI irritation).
- IV: KCl in IV fluids. HIGH-ALERT MEDICATION.

IV POTASSIUM SAFETY RULES:

- NEVER give IV push—can cause fatal arrhythmias
- Maximum concentration: 40 mEq/L in peripheral line; higher concentrations need central line
- Maximum rate: 10-20 mEq/hour (40 mEq/hour with cardiac monitoring in severe cases)
- Always use infusion pump
- Monitor for phlebitis at IV site

Hyperkalemia Signs: Muscle weakness, paresthesias, bradycardia, peaked T waves, widened QRS, cardiac arrest

Hyperkalemia Treatment:

- Calcium gluconate: Cardioprotective (does not lower K+)

- Insulin + glucose: Shifts K+ into cells
- Sodium bicarbonate: Shifts K+ into cells
- Kayexalate (sodium polystyrene sulfonate): Binds K+ in GI tract
- Dialysis: For severe or refractory cases

Clinical Pearl: Calcium gluconate protects the heart but doesn't lower potassium—always follow with therapies that reduce K+.

Sodium

Normal Range: 136-145 mEq/L

Hyponatremia: Confusion, lethargy, seizures, cerebral edema. Causes: SIADH, diuretics, water intoxication.

Treatment: Fluid restriction, treat underlying cause. Severe: 3% saline (slowly—rapid correction causes osmotic demyelination syndrome).

Hypernatremia: Thirst, confusion, lethargy, seizures. Causes: Dehydration, diabetes insipidus.

Treatment: Replace free water (D5W, 0.45% NS). Correct slowly to prevent cerebral edema.

Calcium

Normal Range: 8.5-10.5 mg/dL (ionized: 4.5-5.5 mg/dL)

Hypocalcemia Signs: Tetany, Chvostek's sign, Trousseau's sign, paresthesias, seizures, prolonged QT

Replacement: Calcium gluconate (preferred IV—less irritating) or calcium chloride (more potent but irritating). Oral calcium with vitamin D.

IV Calcium Considerations:

- Give slowly—rapid infusion causes hypotension, bradycardia
- Do NOT mix with bicarbonate (precipitates)
- Monitor for extravasation (tissue necrosis)

Hypercalcemia Signs: "Bones, stones, groans, moans"—bone pain, kidney stones, abdominal pain, confusion/lethargy

Treatment: IV normal saline, loop diuretics, bisphosphonates, calcitonin

Magnesium

Normal Range: 1.5-2.5 mEq/L

Hypomagnesemia Signs: Similar to hypocalcemia—tremors, tetany, seizures, arrhythmias (torsades de pointes)

Replacement: Magnesium sulfate IV or magnesium oxide oral

IV Magnesium Considerations:

- Give slowly—rapid infusion causes flushing, hypotension
- Monitor deep tendon reflexes (absent DTRs = toxicity)
- Have calcium gluconate available as antidote

Uses of Magnesium Sulfate: Eclampsia, torsades de pointes, severe asthma, hypomagnesemia

Magnesium Toxicity: Loss of DTRs, respiratory depression, cardiac arrest. Antidote: calcium gluconate.

Phosphorus

Normal Range: 2.5-4.5 mg/dL

Hypophosphatemia: Muscle weakness, respiratory failure, hemolysis, confusion. Common in refeeding syndrome.

Hyperphosphatemia: Common in CKD. Treat with phosphate binders (calcium acetate, sevelamer, lanthanum).

8.6 Medications for Chronic Kidney Disease

Phosphate Binders

Drugs: Calcium acetate (PhosLo), sevelamer (Renagel), lanthanum (Fosrenol)

Uses: Hyperphosphatemia in CKD

Administration: Take WITH meals (bind dietary phosphate in GI tract)

Sevelamer Advantage: Does not contain calcium (avoids hypercalcemia)

Erythropoiesis-Stimulating Agents (ESAs)

Drugs: Epoetin alfa (Epogen, Procrit), darbepoetin alfa (Aranesp)

Uses: Anemia of CKD, chemotherapy-induced anemia

BLACK BOX WARNINGS:

- Increased risk of cardiovascular events, stroke, death if Hgb > 11 g/dL
- Tumor progression in cancer patients
- Use lowest dose to avoid transfusions

Nursing Considerations:

- Monitor Hgb (target 10-11 g/dL in CKD)
- Ensure adequate iron stores

- Monitor BP (can cause hypertension)
- SubQ or IV administration

Vitamin D Analogues

Drugs: Calcitriol (Rocaltrol), paricalcitol (Zemplar)

Uses: Secondary hyperparathyroidism in CKD, hypocalcemia

Monitoring: Calcium, phosphorus, PTH levels

Calcimimetics

Drug: Cinacalcet (Sensipar)

Uses: Secondary hyperparathyroidism in CKD on dialysis

Mechanism: Increases sensitivity of calcium-sensing receptors → decreases PTH

Adverse Effects: Hypocalcemia (monitor calcium), nausea

8.7 Medications for Urinary Disorders

Urinary Antispasmodics

Drugs: Oxybutynin (Ditropan), tolterodine (Detrol), solifenacin (Vesicare)

Uses: Overactive bladder, urinary urgency/frequency

Mechanism: Anticholinergic—relax bladder smooth muscle

Adverse Effects: Dry mouth, constipation, blurred vision, urinary retention, confusion (especially elderly)

Beers Criteria: Use with caution in elderly due to anticholinergic effects.

Alpha-1 Blockers for BPH

Drugs: Tamsulosin (Flomax), alfuzosin (Uroxatral), doxazosin (Cardura)

Uses: Benign prostatic hyperplasia—relax smooth muscle in prostate and bladder neck

Adverse Effects: Orthostatic hypotension (especially first dose), dizziness, retrograde ejaculation

Nursing Considerations: Take at bedtime. Rise slowly. "First-dose syncope" risk.

5-Alpha Reductase Inhibitors

Drugs: Finasteride (Proscar), dutasteride (Avodart)

Uses: BPH—shrinks prostate over 6-12 months

Adverse Effects: Sexual dysfunction, gynecomastia

PREGNANCY WARNING: Pregnant women should not handle crushed tablets—causes fetal malformations

PSA Monitoring: Decreases PSA by ~50%. Must double reported PSA for accurate interpretation.

8.8 Chapter Summary

- IV Fluids: Isotonic for volume expansion, hypotonic for cellular dehydration, hypertonic for severe hyponatremia.
- Loop Diuretics: Most potent. Cause hypokalemia, ototoxicity. Give IV slowly.
- Thiazides: First-line for HTN. Cause hypokalemia, hypercalcemia.
- K+-Sparing Diuretics: Cause HYPERKALEMIA. Avoid K+ supplements and salt substitutes.
- IV Potassium: HIGH-ALERT. Never IV push. Use infusion pump. Max 10-20 mEq/hr.
- Hyperkalemia Treatment: Calcium gluconate (cardioprotection), insulin+glucose, dialysis.
- ESAs: BLACK BOX—target Hgb 10-11 g/dL. Higher targets increase CV risk.

8.9 Practice Questions

Directions: Select the best answer for each question.

1. A patient with heart failure is receiving furosemide. Which electrolyte should the nurse monitor most closely?

A. Sodium

B. Potassium

C. Calcium

D. Phosphorus

2. A patient is receiving IV potassium chloride. Which finding requires immediate intervention?

A. Potassium level of 3.8 mEq/L

B. Infusion rate of 15 mEq/hour

C. IV push administration ordered

D. Burning sensation at the IV site

3. Which IV fluid is most appropriate for a patient with hypovolemic shock?

A. D5W

B. 0.45% Normal Saline

C. 0.9% Normal Saline or Lactated Ringer's

D. D5 0.45% NS

4. A patient taking spironolactone should avoid:

A. Citrus fruits

B. Potassium-rich foods and salt substitutes

C. Dairy products

D. Green leafy vegetables

5. The nurse should question an order for mannitol in a patient with:

A. Increased intracranial pressure

B. Acute kidney injury with oliguria

C. Heart failure with pulmonary edema

D. Acute glaucoma

6. A patient has a serum sodium of 118 mEq/L. The priority intervention is:

A. Administer 3% saline rapidly

B. Restrict fluids and monitor neurologic status

C. Give normal saline bolus

D. Encourage oral sodium intake

7. Which sign indicates hypocalcemia?

A. Chvostek's sign (facial twitching with tap)

B. Widened QRS complex

C. Depressed deep tendon reflexes

D. Hypertension

8. A patient receiving magnesium sulfate IV has absent deep tendon reflexes. The nurse should:

A. Continue the infusion as ordered

B. Stop the infusion and notify the provider

C. Increase the infusion rate

D. Administer potassium chloride

9. Loop diuretics should be administered slowly via IV to prevent:

A. Hyperkalemia

B. Ototoxicity

C. Hypertension

D. Hyperglycemia

10. Which patient statement indicates understanding of hydrochlorothiazide therapy?

A. I should take this medication at bedtime

B. I should use sunscreen when outdoors

C. I can use salt substitutes freely

D. I should limit my potassium intake

11. A patient with CKD is taking sevelamer (Renagel). The nurse instructs the patient to take this medication:

A. On an empty stomach

B. With meals

C. At bedtime only

D. One hour before meals

12. For a patient with severe hyperkalemia and ECG changes, the first medication to administer is:

A. Sodium polystyrene sulfonate (Kayexalate)

B. Regular insulin with dextrose

C. Calcium gluconate

D. Sodium bicarbonate

13. A patient receiving epoetin alfa (Epogen) should be monitored for:

A. Hypotension

B. Hypertension

C. Bradycardia

D. Hyperkalemia

14. Which IV solution would be most appropriate for a patient with hypernatremia?

A. 0.9% Normal Saline

B. 3% Saline

C. 0.45% Normal Saline

D. Lactated Ringer's

15. A patient taking tamsulosin for BPH should be taught to:

A. Take the medication in the morning with breakfast

B. Rise slowly to prevent dizziness

C. Expect immediate symptom relief

D. Avoid drinking fluids

16. The antidote for magnesium toxicity is:

A. Sodium bicarbonate

B. Potassium chloride

C. Calcium gluconate

D. Naloxone

17. A patient is receiving 0.45% Normal Saline. This solution is classified as:

A. Isotonic

B. Hypotonic

C. Hypertonic

D. Colloid

18. When administering calcium gluconate IV, the nurse should:

A. Give rapid IV push for maximum effect

B. Monitor for bradycardia and hypotension

C. Mix with sodium bicarbonate for compatibility

D. Expect decreased urine output

19. A patient taking finasteride for BPH should understand that:

A. Symptom improvement occurs within days

B. Pregnant women can safely handle the tablets

C. PSA levels may decrease by about 50%

D. The medication increases testosterone levels

20. Which assessment finding indicates effective furosemide therapy in a patient with heart failure?

A. Weight gain of 2 pounds

B. Decreased urine output

C. Resolution of peripheral edema

D. Potassium level of 5.8 mEq/L

CHAPTER 9

Immunologic and Hematologic Medications

9.1 Learning Objectives

By the end of this chapter, you will be able to:

- Differentiate between immunosuppressants and immunostimulants
- Identify the mechanisms and nursing considerations for biologic therapies
- Explain the appropriate use of colony-stimulating factors
- Recognize adverse effects of immunosuppressive therapy
- Apply safety principles for blood product administration
- Describe medications used to treat anemia and coagulation disorders
- Educate patients about immunosuppressive therapy and infection prevention

9.2 Overview of Immunologic and Hematologic Pharmacology

The immune and hematologic systems are closely connected. Immunologic medications modify immune responses—suppressing them in autoimmune diseases and transplant rejection, or stimulating them against cancer. Hematologic medications affect blood cell production, clotting, and oxygen-carrying capacity.

9.3 Immunosuppressants

Calcineurin Inhibitors

Drugs: Cyclosporine (Sandimmune, Neoral), tacrolimus (Prograf)

Mechanism: Inhibit calcineurin → block T-cell activation and IL-2 production

Uses: Organ transplant rejection prevention, autoimmune diseases

NARROW THERAPEUTIC INDEX: Requires drug level monitoring

Adverse Effects:

- NEPHROTOXICITY (major concern)—monitor BUN, creatinine
- Hypertension
- Neurotoxicity (tremor, headache, seizures)

- Hyperglycemia (especially tacrolimus)
- Hyperkalemia
- Increased infection and malignancy risk

Cyclosporine-Specific: Gingival hyperplasia, hirsutism

Drug Interactions: Many! CYP3A4 substrate. Avoid grapefruit juice (increases levels).

Clinical Pearl: Sandimmune and Neoral are NOT interchangeable—different bioavailability.

Antimetabolites

Drugs: Azathioprine (Imuran), mycophenolate (CellCept, Myfortic)

Mechanism: Inhibit purine synthesis → suppress lymphocyte proliferation

Uses: Transplant rejection prevention, autoimmune diseases (lupus, RA)

Adverse Effects:

- Bone marrow suppression (monitor CBC)—leukopenia, thrombocytopenia, anemia
- GI upset (especially mycophenolate)
- Hepatotoxicity (azathioprine)
- Increased infection risk

Azathioprine: Check TPMT enzyme before starting—deficiency increases toxicity. Avoid allopurinol (severe interaction).

Mycophenolate: BLACK BOX WARNING for pregnancy—causes birth defects. Effective contraception required.

mTOR Inhibitors

Drugs: Sirolimus (Rapamune), everolimus (Zortress)

Mechanism: Inhibit mTOR pathway → block T-cell and B-cell activation

Uses: Transplant rejection prevention, often with calcineurin inhibitors

Adverse Effects: Hyperlipidemia, thrombocytopenia, impaired wound healing, mouth ulcers, pneumonitis

Advantage: Less nephrotoxic than calcineurin inhibitors

Corticosteroids

Drugs: Prednisone, methylprednisolone, dexamethasone

Uses in Immunosuppression: Transplant (induction and maintenance), autoimmune diseases, acute rejection episodes

[See Chapter 5 for detailed corticosteroid information]

9.4 Biologic Response Modifiers

TNF-Alpha Inhibitors

Drugs: Infliximab (Remicade), adalimumab (Humira), etanercept (Enbrel), golimumab (Simponi), certolizumab (Cimzia)

Mechanism: Block tumor necrosis factor-alpha → reduce inflammation

Uses: Rheumatoid arthritis, psoriatic arthritis, ankylosing spondylitis, Crohn's disease, ulcerative colitis, psoriasis

BLACK BOX WARNINGS:

- Serious infections including TB, invasive fungal infections—screen for TB before starting
- Lymphoma and other malignancies

Other Adverse Effects: Injection site reactions, infusion reactions, hepatotoxicity, heart failure exacerbation, demyelinating disorders

Nursing Considerations:

- TB skin test or IGRA before initiation
- Monitor for signs of infection
- Do not give live vaccines during therapy
- Teach self-injection technique if applicable

Clinical Pearl: Hold TNF inhibitors before surgery and during active infection.

Interleukin Inhibitors

IL-1 Inhibitors: Anakinra (Kineret)—RA, autoinflammatory diseases

IL-6 Inhibitors: Tocilizumab (Actemra), sarilumab (Kevzara)—RA, cytokine release syndrome

IL-17 Inhibitors: Secukinumab (Cosentyx), ixekizumab (Taltz)—psoriasis, psoriatic arthritis

IL-12/23 Inhibitors: Ustekinumab (Stelara)—psoriasis, Crohn's disease

Common Concerns: Infection risk, injection site reactions, monitor CBC and LFTs

B-Cell Targeting Agents

Rituximab (Rituxan):

- Mechanism: Anti-CD20 monoclonal antibody—depletes B cells
- Uses: Non-Hodgkin lymphoma, CLL, RA, granulomatosis with polyangiitis

- BLACK BOX WARNINGS: Fatal infusion reactions, severe mucocutaneous reactions, hepatitis B reactivation, PML
- Premedicate with acetaminophen, diphenhydramine, and corticosteroid

T-Cell Targeting Agents

Abatacept (Orencia): Blocks T-cell co-stimulation. Used for RA.

9.5 Immunostimulants

Interferons

Interferon alfa: Hepatitis B and C, certain cancers

Interferon beta: Multiple sclerosis (reduces relapse rate)

Adverse Effects: Flu-like symptoms (fever, myalgia, fatigue), depression, bone marrow suppression, hepatotoxicity

Nursing Considerations: Give at bedtime to sleep through flu-like symptoms. Premedicate with acetaminophen.

Colony-Stimulating Factors

Filgrastim (Neupogen), pegfilgrastim (Neulasta): G-CSF—stimulates neutrophil production

- Uses: Chemotherapy-induced neutropenia, stem cell mobilization
- Adverse Effects: Bone pain (common), splenomegaly, ARDS (rare)
- Timing: Give 24 hours after chemotherapy, not within 24 hours before

Sargramostim (Leukine): GM-CSF—stimulates multiple cell lines

Oprelvekin (Neumega): IL-11—stimulates platelet production. Discontinued but may appear on exams.

9.6 Vaccines and Immunoglobulins

Vaccines

Live Attenuated: MMR, varicella, rotavirus, intranasal flu, yellow fever

- CONTRAINDICATED in immunocompromised patients and pregnancy

Inactivated/Killed: Flu (injection), hepatitis A and B, polio (IPV), rabies

Toxoid: Tetanus, diphtheria

mRNA: COVID-19 vaccines (Pfizer, Moderna)

Nursing Considerations: Screen for allergies, contraindications. Have epinephrine available. Observe for 15-30 minutes after administration.

Immunoglobulins

IVIG (Intravenous Immunoglobulin):

- Uses: Primary immunodeficiency, ITP, Guillain-Barré, Kawasaki disease
- Adverse Effects: Infusion reactions, headache, renal dysfunction, thrombosis
- Infuse slowly initially, monitor vital signs

Specific Immunoglobulins: RhoGAM (Rh incompatibility), hepatitis B Ig, rabies Ig, tetanus Ig, varicella-zoster Ig

9.7 Medications for Anemia

Iron Preparations

Oral Iron: Ferrous sulfate, ferrous gluconate, ferrous fumarate

Administration:

- Take on empty stomach for best absorption (with food if GI upset)
- Take with vitamin C (enhances absorption)
- Avoid with antacids, dairy, tea, coffee (decrease absorption)
- Separate from fluoroquinolones, tetracyclines, levothyroxine by 2 hours

Adverse Effects: GI upset, constipation, black stools (normal)

IV Iron: Iron sucrose (Venofer), ferric carboxymaltose (Injectafer), iron dextran

- Iron dextran: Test dose required—anaphylaxis risk
- Monitor for infusion reactions

Clinical Pearl: Liquid iron can stain teeth—use straw and rinse mouth after.

Vitamin B12 and Folic Acid

Cyanocobalamin (B12): For pernicious anemia, B12 deficiency

- Often requires IM injection (oral not absorbed in pernicious anemia)
- Lifelong therapy if intrinsic factor deficiency

Folic Acid: For folate deficiency, pregnancy, methotrexate therapy

- IMPORTANT: Do not give folic acid alone if B12 deficiency suspected—can mask B12 deficiency and cause neurologic damage

Erythropoiesis-Stimulating Agents

[See Chapter 8 for ESA details]

9.8 Anticoagulants, Antiplatelets, and Thrombolytics

[See Chapter 2 for detailed coverage of anticoagulants and antiplatelets]

Thrombolytics (Fibrinolytics)

Drugs: Alteplase (tPA, Activase), reteplase (Retavase), tenecteplase (TNKase)

Mechanism: Convert plasminogen to plasmin → dissolve clots

Uses: Acute MI (within 12 hours), acute ischemic stroke (within 3-4.5 hours), massive PE

MAJOR RISK: BLEEDING—can be life-threatening

Contraindications:

- Recent surgery, trauma, or invasive procedures
- Active internal bleeding
- History of hemorrhagic stroke
- Severe uncontrolled hypertension
- Intracranial neoplasm, AVM, aneurysm

Nursing Considerations:

- Monitor for bleeding—neuro checks, puncture sites, urine, stool
- Avoid unnecessary venipunctures and invasive procedures
- Have aminocaproic acid available (antidote for fibrinolysis)
- Monitor vital signs frequently

9.9 Hemostatic Agents

Aminocaproic Acid (Amicar)

Mechanism: Inhibits fibrinolysis → promotes clot stability

Uses: Bleeding from fibrinolysis, post-surgical bleeding, hemophilia adjunct

Vitamin K (Phytonadione)

Uses: Warfarin reversal, vitamin K deficiency, newborn prophylaxis

Administration: Oral preferred. IV only for severe bleeding (give slowly—anaphylaxis risk).

[See Chapter 2 for warfarin reversal details]

Desmopressin (DDAVP)

Uses: Mild hemophilia A, von Willebrand disease—increases factor VIII and vWF release

Administration: IV, SubQ, or intranasal

Clotting Factor Concentrates

Factor VIII: Hemophilia A

Factor IX: Hemophilia B

[These are blood products with specific handling and administration requirements]

9.10 Blood Products

Packed Red Blood Cells (PRBCs)

Indications: Symptomatic anemia, acute blood loss

Administration:

- ABO and Rh compatibility required
- Use blood administration set with filter
- Infuse within 4 hours
- Only compatible IV solution: 0.9% NS

Platelets

Indications: Thrombocytopenia, platelet dysfunction, active bleeding

Administration: Infuse rapidly (30-60 minutes). ABO compatibility preferred but not required.

Fresh Frozen Plasma (FFP)

Indications: Coagulation factor deficiency, warfarin reversal, massive transfusion, DIC

Administration: Must be ABO compatible. Thaw before use.

Transfusion Reactions

Acute Hemolytic Reaction: ABO incompatibility. Fever, chills, flank pain, hemoglobinuria, hypotension. STOP TRANSFUSION IMMEDIATELY.

Febrile Non-Hemolytic: Most common. Fever, chills. Stop transfusion, give antipyretics, may resume slowly.

Allergic Reaction: Urticaria, pruritus, anaphylaxis (rare). Stop transfusion, give antihistamine/epinephrine.

TRALI (Transfusion-Related Acute Lung Injury): Respiratory distress, hypoxia, bilateral infiltrates within 6 hours. Supportive care.

Volume Overload (TACO): Dyspnea, hypertension, jugular distension. Slow or stop transfusion, diuretics.

Nursing Actions for Reaction:

- STOP the transfusion immediately
- Keep IV line open with NS
- Notify provider and blood bank
- Monitor vital signs
- Send blood bag and tubing to lab
- Document everything

9.11 Medications for Sickle Cell Disease

Hydroxyurea: Increases fetal hemoglobin production → reduces sickling and crises

- Monitor CBC—bone marrow suppression
- Teratogenic—contraception required

L-glutamine (Endari): Reduces oxidative stress in RBCs. Oral powder.

Voxelotor (Oxbryta): Stabilizes hemoglobin → reduces sickling.

Crizanlizumab (Adakveo): Blocks cell adhesion → reduces vaso-occlusive crises.

9.12 Chapter Summary

- Calcineurin Inhibitors (cyclosporine, tacrolimus): Narrow TI. Monitor levels, nephrotoxicity, BP, glucose.
- TNF Inhibitors: Screen for TB before starting. BLACK BOX for infections and malignancy.
- Colony-Stimulating Factors: Give 24 hours after chemo. Bone pain common.
- Oral Iron: Take on empty stomach with vitamin C. Black stools expected.
- B12 vs Folate: Never give folate alone if B12 deficiency possible.
- Thrombolytics: Major bleeding risk. Many contraindications. Monitor neuro status.
- Transfusion Reactions: STOP transfusion, maintain IV access, notify provider.

9.13 Practice Questions

Directions: Select the best answer for each question.

1. Before starting infliximab (Remicade), the nurse should ensure:

A. Hepatitis C screening is complete

B. TB screening is complete

C. HIV testing is done

D. Pregnancy test is negative

2. A patient taking tacrolimus has a tremor and elevated creatinine. The nurse recognizes these as signs of:

A. Therapeutic drug effect

B. Drug toxicity

C. Allergic reaction

D. Infection

3. A patient receiving filgrastim (Neupogen) reports severe bone pain. The nurse should:

A. Recognize this as an expected side effect

B. Stop the medication immediately

C. Notify the provider of an allergic reaction

D. Administer calcium supplements

4. Which instruction is most important for a patient taking oral iron supplements?

A. Take with antacids to reduce GI upset

B. Take on an empty stomach with orange juice

C. Take with dairy products for better absorption

D. Take at the same time as thyroid medication

5. A patient is receiving a blood transfusion and develops fever, chills, and flank pain. The priority action is:

A. Slow the transfusion rate

B. Administer acetaminophen and continue

C. Stop the transfusion immediately

D. Notify the provider and continue the transfusion

6. A patient on cyclosporine should avoid:

A. Green leafy vegetables

B. Grapefruit juice

C. Dairy products

D. High-protein foods

7. The nurse should question an order for a live vaccine in a patient taking:

A. Acetaminophen

B. Prednisone 40 mg daily for 3 weeks

C. Ibuprofen

D. Ferrous sulfate

8. A patient with pernicious anemia requires B12 administration via:

A. Oral tablets

B. Sublingual route

C. Intramuscular injection

D. Topical patch

9. Which finding indicates an adverse effect of azathioprine therapy?

A. Increased appetite

B. WBC count of 2,500/mcL

C. Weight gain

D. Elevated blood glucose

10. Alteplase (tPA) is contraindicated in a patient with:

A. Diabetes mellitus

B. Recent hemorrhagic stroke

C. History of MI

D. Hypertension controlled with medication

11. A patient receiving rituximab develops difficulty breathing and hypotension during the infusion. The nurse should:

A. Slow the infusion and monitor closely

B. Stop the infusion and initiate emergency care

C. Continue the infusion with supplemental oxygen

D. Administer an antihistamine and continue

12. The nurse is teaching a patient about mycophenolate (CellCept). Which statement requires clarification?

A. I will avoid becoming pregnant while on this medication

B. I should report signs of infection promptly

C. I can take this medication with antacids

D. I may experience nausea and diarrhea

13. When administering IV iron dextran, the nurse should first:

A. Infuse rapidly to minimize reactions

B. Administer a test dose

C. Mix with D5W

D. Give via IV push

14. A patient with hemophilia A is scheduled for dental surgery. The nurse anticipates administration of:

A. Vitamin K

B. Factor VIII concentrate

C. Fresh frozen plasma

D. Aminocaproic acid alone

15. Which adverse effect is most concerning in a patient on interferon therapy?

A. Flu-like symptoms

B. Injection site redness

C. Depression and suicidal ideation

D. Mild fatigue

16. A nurse is preparing to administer PRBCs. The only compatible IV solution is:

A. D5W

B. Lactated Ringer's

C. 0.9% Normal Saline

D. D5 0.45% NS

17. A patient taking hydroxyurea for sickle cell disease should be monitored for:

A. Hyperglycemia

B. Bone marrow suppression

C. Renal toxicity

D. Hepatomegaly

18. The antidote for thrombolytic-induced bleeding is:

A. Protamine sulfate

B. Vitamin K

C. Aminocaproic acid

D. Fresh frozen plasma alone

19. A patient receiving IVIG reports severe headache. The nurse should:

A. Reassure that this is a common side effect

B. Slow the infusion rate and monitor

C. Continue the infusion as ordered

D. Administer aspirin for pain

20. Which patient statement indicates understanding of TNF inhibitor therapy?

A. I should receive my annual flu shot as usual

B. I will report any signs of infection immediately

C. I can stop the medication when I feel better

D. This medication will cure my rheumatoid arthritis

CHAPTER 10

Special Populations and High-Alert Medications

10.1 Learning Objectives

By the end of this chapter, you will be able to:

- Apply pharmacokinetic principles to pediatric medication administration
- Identify medications requiring dose adjustment in geriatric patients
- Explain the FDA pregnancy risk categories and safe medication use during pregnancy
- Recognize high-alert medications and implement safety strategies
- Apply the principles of medication reconciliation
- Describe strategies to prevent medication errors
- Educate special populations about medication safety

10.2 Overview

Certain patient populations require special consideration when administering medications. Age, pregnancy, lactation, and organ function all affect how drugs are processed. Additionally, some medications carry such high risk that they require extra safety measures. This chapter integrates concepts from previous chapters with a focus on vulnerable populations and error prevention.

10.3 Pediatric Pharmacology

Pharmacokinetic Differences in Children

Absorption:

- Gastric pH higher in neonates (less acidic) → affects drug absorption
- Decreased gastric emptying time in infants
- Greater skin permeability → increased topical absorption
- IM absorption variable (less muscle mass, unpredictable blood flow)

Distribution:

- Higher percentage of body water → larger volume of distribution for water-soluble drugs
- Lower plasma protein binding → more free (active) drug

- Immature blood-brain barrier → CNS drugs may have enhanced effects

Metabolism:

- Immature hepatic enzymes in neonates → slower drug metabolism
- Children 1-12 years may have FASTER metabolism than adults

Excretion:

- Immature renal function in neonates → slower drug elimination
- Adult renal function reached by age 1-2 years

Pediatric Dosing Principles

Weight-Based Dosing: Most pediatric doses calculated as mg/kg

- Always verify weight in kilograms
- Double-check calculations
- Use appropriate measuring devices (oral syringes, not household spoons)

Body Surface Area (BSA): Used for chemotherapy and some critical medications

Maximum Dose: Calculated pediatric dose should not exceed adult dose

Clinical Pearl: A 10-fold dosing error is the most common and dangerous pediatric medication error. Always question doses that seem too high or too low.

High-Risk Medications in Pediatrics

- Opioids—respiratory depression risk higher
- Sedatives—paradoxical reactions possible
- Insulin—hypoglycemia risk
- Anticonvulsants—narrow therapeutic index
- Digoxin—toxicity risk
- Chemotherapy—weight-based calculations critical

Medications to Avoid in Pediatrics

- Aspirin: Reye syndrome risk in viral illness (< 19 years)
- Tetracyclines: Tooth discoloration, bone effects (< 8 years)
- Fluoroquinolones: Cartilage damage (use only when no alternatives)
- Codeine: FDA contraindicated < 12 years (respiratory depression)
- Promethazine: BLACK BOX < 2 years (respiratory depression)

- OTC cough/cold medications: Not recommended < 4 years

10.4 Geriatric Pharmacology

Pharmacokinetic Changes with Aging

Absorption:

- Decreased gastric acid → may affect drug dissolution
- Decreased GI motility → delayed absorption
- Generally minor clinical impact

Distribution:

- Decreased total body water → higher concentration of water-soluble drugs
- Increased body fat → prolonged effects of fat-soluble drugs (benzodiazepines, opioids)
- Decreased albumin → more free drug (toxicity risk)

Metabolism:

- Decreased hepatic blood flow and liver mass
- Reduced Phase I metabolism (oxidation)
- Prolonged drug half-life

Excretion:

- Decreased renal blood flow and GFR
- Reduced drug clearance → accumulation risk
- Creatinine may appear normal despite reduced function (less muscle mass)

Clinical Pearl: "Start low and go slow"—begin with lower doses and titrate gradually in elderly patients.

Beers Criteria

Definition: AGS Beers Criteria lists potentially inappropriate medications (PIMs) for older adults

Categories:

- Medications to avoid in most older adults
- Medications to avoid in certain conditions
- Medications to use with caution
- Drug-drug interactions to avoid

Common Beers Criteria Medications to Avoid

Anticholinergics:

- First-generation antihistamines (diphenhydramine)
- Tricyclic antidepressants (amitriptyline)
- Antispasmodics (oxybutynin, dicyclomine)
- Risks: Confusion, falls, urinary retention, constipation

Benzodiazepines:

- All benzodiazepines (long and short-acting)
- Risks: Sedation, falls, fractures, cognitive impairment

Sedative-Hypnotics:

- Zolpidem, eszopiclone
- Risks: Falls, delirium, complex sleep behaviors

Other PIMs:

- NSAIDs (GI bleeding, renal, cardiovascular risks)
- Muscle relaxants (carisoprodol, cyclobenzaprine)
- Meperidine (neurotoxic metabolite)
- Sliding scale insulin alone (hypoglycemia risk)
- Sulfonylureas (long-acting: glyburide—hypoglycemia)

Polypharmacy

Definition: Use of multiple medications, often defined as $\geq$ 5 medications

Risks:

- Drug-drug interactions
- Adverse drug reactions
- Medication non-adherence
- Increased falls and hospitalizations

Nursing Interventions:

- Medication reconciliation at every encounter
- "Brown bag" reviews—have patient bring all medications
- Identify and discontinue unnecessary medications
- Simplify regimens when possible

10.5 Pregnancy and Lactation

FDA Pregnancy Categories (Legacy System)

[Note: FDA now uses narrative labeling (PLLR) instead of letter categories, but categories may still appear on exams]

- Category A: Controlled studies show no risk
- Category B: No evidence of risk in humans (animal studies negative or no human studies)
- Category C: Risk cannot be ruled out (use if benefit > risk)
- Category D: Positive evidence of risk (use if benefit > risk in serious conditions)
- Category X: CONTRAINDICATED—risks clearly outweigh benefits

Teratogenic Medications (Category X or Contraindicated)

- Isotretinoin (Accutane): Severe birth defects—iPLEDGE program required
- Methotrexate: Fetal death, congenital malformations
- Warfarin: Fetal warfarin syndrome (first trimester), CNS abnormalities
- Statins: Fetal harm
- ACE inhibitors/ARBs: Fetal renal damage, oligohydramnios (contraindicated all trimesters)
- Valproic acid: Neural tube defects, developmental delays
- Phenytoin: Fetal hydantoin syndrome
- Lithium: Ebstein's anomaly (cardiac defect)—Category D, not X, but avoid if possible
- Thalidomide: Limb defects
- Misoprostol: Uterine contractions, abortion

Safer Medication Options in Pregnancy

- Pain: Acetaminophen (preferred)
- Nausea: Pyridoxine (B6), doxylamine, ondansetron
- Antibiotics: Penicillins, cephalosporins, azithromycin (generally safe)
- Depression: SSRIs (benefits often outweigh risks; paroxetine has concerns)
- Anticoagulation: Heparin, LMWH (do not cross placenta)
- Diabetes: Insulin (does not cross placenta)
- Hypertension: Labetalol, methyldopa, nifedipine

Lactation Considerations

- Most drugs transfer into breast milk to some degree
- Infant dose usually < 10% of maternal dose
- Resources: LactMed database (NIH) for current information

Contraindicated in Breastfeeding:

- Chemotherapy agents
- Radioactive compounds
- Drugs of abuse
- Some anticonvulsants, lithium (monitor infant)

10.6 Renal and Hepatic Impairment

Renal Impairment

Impact: Reduced drug excretion → accumulation, prolonged effects, toxicity

Drugs Requiring Adjustment:

- Aminoglycosides, vancomycin
- Digoxin
- Metformin (contraindicated if eGFR < 30)
- DOACs (dose adjustment or avoidance)
- Gabapentin, pregabalin
- Many antibiotics

Nursing Considerations:

- Check renal function (eGFR, CrCl) before and during therapy
- Verify dose adjustments in drug references
- Monitor for drug accumulation and toxicity

Hepatic Impairment

Impact: Reduced drug metabolism → accumulation, prolonged effects

Drugs Requiring Caution:

- Opioids (increased sedation, encephalopathy risk)
- Benzodiazepines (use lorazepam, oxazepam—no active metabolites)
- Acetaminophen (hepatotoxic—lower max dose)
- Statins (monitor LFTs)

- Warfarin (decreased clotting factor synthesis)

Nursing Considerations:

- Assess liver function (AST, ALT, bilirubin, albumin)
- Monitor for signs of toxicity and encephalopathy
- Many drugs have no specific hepatic dosing—use clinical judgment

10.7 High-Alert Medications

Definition: Medications that bear heightened risk of causing significant patient harm when used in error

[ISMP maintains the High-Alert Medications list]

ISMP High-Alert Medication Categories

- Anticoagulants (heparin, warfarin, DOACs)
- Insulin
- Opioids
- Neuromuscular blocking agents
- Chemotherapy
- Concentrated electrolytes (potassium chloride, sodium chloride > 0.9%)
- IV adrenergic agonists and antagonists
- Dialysis solutions
- Epidural and intrathecal medications

Safety Strategies for High-Alert Medications

Independent Double Checks: Two nurses independently verify:

- Right patient, drug, dose, route, time
- Calculations (especially weight-based)
- Pump programming

Standardization:

- Standardized concentrations
- Premixed solutions when available
- Limit variety of concentrations available

Technology:

- Smart pumps with drug libraries

- Barcode medication administration (BCMA)
- Clinical decision support systems

Storage:

- Separate high-alert medications from look-alike drugs
- Use warning labels and auxiliary stickers
- Remove concentrated electrolytes from patient care areas

10.8 Look-Alike/Sound-Alike (LASA) Medications

[ISMP maintains LASA drug list with tall-man lettering]

Common LASA Pairs:

- hydrALAZINE vs. hydrOXYzine
- predniSONE vs. prednisoLONE
- DOPamine vs. DOBUTamine
- vinCRIStine vs. vinBLAStine
- EPINEPHrine vs. ePHEDrine
- metFORMIN vs. metroNIDAZOLE
- LaMICtal vs. LamiSIL

Prevention Strategies:

- Use both generic and brand names
- Include indication on prescription
- Implement tall-man lettering
- Use barcode scanning
- Store LASA drugs separately

10.9 Medication Reconciliation

Definition: Process of comparing a patient's medication orders to all medications the patient has been taking

When to Perform:

- Admission to any healthcare facility
- Transfers between units or facilities
- Discharge
- Outpatient visits (especially after hospitalization)

What to Include:

- Prescription medications
- Over-the-counter medications
- Vitamins and supplements
- Herbal products
- Vaccines

Goals:

- Identify discrepancies
- Prevent omissions and duplications
- Ensure medication appropriateness
- Communicate accurate medication list

10.10 Medication Error Prevention

The Rights of Medication Administration

- Right Patient—verify with two identifiers
- Right Drug—check label three times
- Right Dose—verify calculation, question unusual doses
- Right Route—confirm appropriateness
- Right Time—within scheduled window
- Right Documentation—document after administration
- Right Reason—understand why patient is receiving medication
- Right Response—monitor for expected/adverse effects

Common Causes of Medication Errors

- Illegible handwriting (use CPOE)
- Verbal orders (read back and verify)
- Abbreviations (avoid dangerous abbreviations)
- Calculation errors (always double-check)
- Similar drug names
- Interruptions during medication administration
- Inadequate patient monitoring

Do Not Use Abbreviations (TJC)

- U (unit)—write "unit"
- IU (international unit)—write "international unit"
- Q.D., QD, q.d., qd (daily)—write "daily"
- Q.O.D., QOD (every other day)—write "every other day"
- Trailing zero (X.0 mg)—write "X mg"
- Lack of leading zero (.X mg)—write "0.X mg"
- MS, MSO4, MgSO4—write "morphine sulfate" or "magnesium sulfate"

10.11 Patient Education Principles

Teach-Back Method: Ask patient to explain in their own words what they learned

Key Teaching Points:

- Name and purpose of medication
- How and when to take it
- Expected effects and side effects
- What to report to provider
- Storage requirements
- Refill information

Health Literacy Considerations:

- Use plain language
- Limit information to 3-5 key points
- Use visual aids when appropriate
- Provide written instructions

10.12 Chapter Summary

- Pediatrics: Weight-based dosing. Avoid aspirin (Reye), tetracyclines (< 8 yr), codeine (< 12 yr).
- Geriatrics: "Start low, go slow." Beers Criteria identifies PIMs. Avoid anticholinergics, benzodiazepines.
- Pregnancy: Category X drugs contraindicated. Avoid ACE inhibitors, warfarin, isotretinoin, valproic acid.
- Renal/Hepatic: Adjust doses for impaired excretion/metabolism. Monitor for toxicity.
- High-Alert Meds: Independent double checks, standardization, smart pumps, proper storage.
- LASA Drugs: Use tall-man lettering, both names, barcode scanning.

- Med Reconciliation: Perform at all transitions of care. Include ALL medications and supplements.

10.13 Practice Questions

Directions: Select the best answer for each question.

1. A nurse is calculating a pediatric medication dose. Which action is most important?

A. Use the adult dose divided by age

B. Verify the child's weight in kilograms

C. Estimate the dose based on the child's appearance

D. Use the same dose as for older children

2. An 82-year-old patient is prescribed diphenhydramine for sleep. The nurse should:

A. Administer as prescribed

B. Question the order based on Beers Criteria

C. Suggest increasing the dose for effectiveness

D. Give with a sedative for better results

3. Which medication is contraindicated throughout pregnancy?

A. Acetaminophen

B. Penicillin

C. ACE inhibitors

D. Ondansetron

4. A nurse is administering insulin. Which safety practice is essential?

A. Administer without verification to save time

B. Have another nurse independently verify the dose

C. Round the dose to the nearest whole number

D. Use any available syringe for measurement

5. The nurse identifies hydrALAZINE and hydrOXYzine stored next to each other. The appropriate action is:

A. Leave them together as they are similar

B. Separate them to prevent medication errors

C. Combine them in one container

D. Report the pharmacy for incorrect labeling

6. Which patient requires dose adjustment for renal impairment?

A. Patient on lisinopril with normal creatinine

B. Patient on metformin with eGFR of 25 mL/min

C. Patient on acetaminophen with normal renal function

D. Patient on levothyroxine with mild CKD

7. A pregnant patient asks about taking ibuprofen for back pain. The nurse should advise:

A. Ibuprofen is safe throughout pregnancy

B. Use acetaminophen instead

C. Take ibuprofen only in the third trimester

D. NSAIDs are preferred in pregnancy

8. An elderly patient is taking 12 medications. The priority nursing intervention is:

A. Add more medications to address side effects

B. Perform comprehensive medication reconciliation

C. Assume all medications are necessary

D. Discontinue all medications

9. Which abbreviation should NEVER be used in medication orders?

A. mg

B. mL

C. U (for unit)

D. tab

10. A medication error occurs. The nurse's first action should be:

A. Hide the error to avoid punishment

B. Assess the patient for harm

C. Blame the pharmacy

D. Complete an incident report before assessment

11. When performing medication reconciliation at discharge, the nurse should include:

A. Only new prescriptions from hospitalization

B. Only prescription medications

C. All medications including OTC, vitamins, and supplements

D. Only medications that changed during admission

12. A child with a viral illness should NOT receive:

A. Acetaminophen

B. Ibuprofen

C. Aspirin

D. Oral rehydration solution

13. Which statement about geriatric pharmacokinetics is correct?

A. Drug metabolism is faster in elderly patients

B. Decreased renal function prolongs drug elimination

C. Elderly patients need higher doses of most medications

D. Body fat decreases with age in most patients

14. The nurse is preparing concentrated potassium chloride for IV infusion. The correct action is:

A. Give by IV push for faster effect

B. Use premixed solutions when available

C. Store at the bedside for convenience

D. Administer without a pump

15. A patient taking warfarin becomes pregnant. The nurse anticipates:

A. Continuing warfarin throughout pregnancy

B. Switching to heparin or LMWH

C. Increasing the warfarin dose

D. Adding aspirin to the regimen

16. Which is a characteristic of high-alert medications?

A. They are used infrequently

B. They have low potential for patient harm

C. They require additional safety measures

D. They can be administered without verification

17. A 7-year-old needs an antibiotic for a respiratory infection. Which medication should the nurse question?

A. Amoxicillin

B. Azithromycin

C. Doxycycline

D. Cephalexin

18. The teach-back method involves:

A. Reading instructions to the patient repeatedly

B. Asking the patient to explain what they learned

C. Teaching only family members

D. Providing written materials without discussion

19. An elderly patient on multiple medications develops confusion. The nurse should first consider:

A. This is normal aging

B. Possible adverse drug reaction

C. Need for additional sedation

D. Psychiatric consultation

20. Which safety strategy is most effective for preventing high-alert medication errors?

A. Relying on memory alone

B. Independent double checks by two nurses

C. Skipping verification when busy

D. Using any available concentration

Answer Key and Rationales

Chapter 1: Foundations of Pharmacology

1. Answer: C — Hepatic metabolism of medications

Rationale: Liver cirrhosis impairs hepatic function, reducing the liver's ability to metabolize medications, leading to accumulation and toxicity risk.

2. Answer: B — Decrease the anticoagulant effect of warfarin

Rationale: Rifampin is a potent CYP450 inducer, increasing warfarin metabolism and decreasing its effect. INR will likely decrease.

3. Answer: C — There is a small margin between therapeutic and toxic dose

Rationale: Narrow therapeutic index means little margin between effective and toxic doses. Digoxin range is 0.5-2.0 ng/mL.

4. Answer: B — After one half-life, half will be eliminated from my body

Rationale: Half-life is the time for plasma concentration to decrease by 50%. It takes 4-5 half-lives for near-complete elimination.

5. Answer: A — Absorption

Rationale: Levothyroxine absorption is affected by food, especially calcium, iron, and fiber. Empty stomach maximizes absorption.

6. Answer: B — Additive interaction

Rationale: Warfarin and aspirin together have additive effects on bleeding risk—warfarin inhibits clotting factors, aspirin inhibits platelets.

7. Answer: B — Consider it may be an adverse drug reaction

Rationale: New confusion in older adults on new medications should always raise ADR suspicion. Never assume it's just aging.

8. Answer: B — Increased phenytoin levels and toxicity

Rationale: CYP450 inhibitors slow phenytoin metabolism, causing accumulation. Phenytoin has a narrow TI, so toxicity occurs quickly.

9. Answer: C — 78-year-old on eight medications

Rationale: Advanced age, multiple conditions, and polypharmacy are major ADR risk factors.

10. Answer: B — IV meds bypass the first-pass effect completely

Rationale: IV administration goes directly into circulation—100% bioavailability, no first-pass metabolism.

11. Answer: B — Have a narrow therapeutic index

Rationale: Aminoglycosides have narrow TI. Peak levels ensure efficacy; trough levels prevent toxicity (nephro/ototoxicity).

12. Answer: B — Inhibiting intestinal CYP3A4 enzymes

Rationale: Grapefruit juice inhibits intestinal CYP3A4, allowing more drug absorption and higher blood levels.

13. Answer: B — Oral contraceptives

Rationale: St. John's Wort induces CYP450, reducing oral contraceptive effectiveness and risking pregnancy.

14. Answer: C — A Type I hypersensitivity reaction

Rationale: Immediate hives and breathing difficulty = Type I (IgE-mediated) reaction. Can progress to anaphylaxis.

15. Answer: B — Child's weight in kilograms

Rationale: Pediatric doses are calculated by weight (mg/kg) to ensure appropriate levels.

16. Answer: C — Drugs excreted primarily by the kidneys

Rationale: CKD impairs renal excretion, causing accumulation of renally excreted drugs like aminoglycosides, vancomycin, digoxin.

17. Answer: B — Respiratory depression

Rationale: Opioids + benzodiazepines = additive CNS/respiratory depression. FDA black box warning exists for this combination.

18. Answer: B — Steady state occurs when intake equals elimination

Rationale: Steady state achieved when drug administration rate equals elimination rate. Occurs after 4-5 half-lives.

19. Answer: B — Provide more consistent blood levels with less frequent dosing

Rationale: Extended-release provides consistent levels with less frequent dosing. Never crush—destroys the mechanism.

20. Answer: B — Include over-the-counter medications and supplements

Rationale: Complete reconciliation includes all substances: prescriptions, OTC, vitamins, supplements, herbals.

Chapter 2: Cardiovascular Medications

1. Answer: B — Accumulation of bradykinin

Rationale: ACE inhibitors block bradykinin breakdown, causing accumulation that irritates airways and causes persistent dry cough.

2. Answer: B — Apical heart rate

Rationale: Beta blockers slow heart rate. Check apical pulse and hold if HR < 60 bpm.

3. Answer: B — Hold the digoxin and notify the provider

Rationale: Hypokalemia (K+ 3.0) significantly increases digoxin toxicity risk. Hold and notify provider.

4. Answer: B — aPTT

Rationale: Heparin effectiveness is monitored with aPTT (goal 1.5-2.5 × control).

5. Answer: B — Maintain consistent intake of vitamin K foods

Rationale: Patients should maintain CONSISTENT vitamin K intake—not avoid it—for stable INR.

6. Answer: D — I can take this with my sildenafil if pain is severe

Rationale: NEVER combine nitrates with PDE5 inhibitors (sildenafil)—causes severe, potentially fatal hypotension.

7. Answer: A — Administer over at least 1-2 minutes

Rationale: Rapid IV push of furosemide can cause ototoxicity. Administer slowly over 1-2 minutes.

8. Answer: A — Pulmonary toxicity

Rationale: Amiodarone causes pulmonary fibrosis, hepatotoxicity, thyroid dysfunction. Monitor chest X-ray and pulmonary function.

9. Answer: C — Tell all healthcare providers you take this medication

Rationale: Antiplatelet therapy affects bleeding risk. All providers must know for procedures and medication decisions.

10. Answer: C — Notify the provider immediately

Rationale: Muscle pain on statins may indicate myopathy/rhabdomyolysis—potentially life-threatening. Requires immediate evaluation.

11. Answer: B — Holding warfarin and monitoring for bleeding

Rationale: INR 4.5 is supratherapeutic with high bleeding risk. Hold warfarin and monitor closely.

12. Answer: B — Anorexia

Rationale: Anorexia (loss of appetite) is often the FIRST sign of digoxin toxicity, before cardiac symptoms.

13. Answer: B — Hypokalemia

Rationale: Furosemide causes hypokalemia, which significantly increases digoxin toxicity risk. Monitor K+ closely.

14. Answer: C — Inject into the abdomen, rotating sites

Rationale: Enoxaparin: Inject deep SubQ in abdomen, rotate sites. Do NOT expel air bubble. Do NOT rub site.

15. Answer: C — I should not crush this medication

Rationale: DOACs should not be crushed—alters drug release. They don't require routine lab monitoring like warfarin.

16. Answer: C — New onset of ankle swelling

Rationale: Peripheral edema (ankle swelling) is a common adverse effect of dihydropyridine CCBs like amlodipine.

17. Answer: B — To prevent development of tolerance

Rationale: A nitrate-free period (10-12 hours, usually overnight) prevents tolerance development.

18. Answer: C — Patient with asthma and wheezing

Rationale: Beta blockers cause bronchospasm—contraindicated in asthma. This patient should not receive beta blockers.

19. Answer: B — Bleeding

Rationale: tPA is a thrombolytic that dissolves clots. Bleeding is the major risk requiring close monitoring.

20. Answer: B — Potassium-rich foods and salt substitutes

Rationale: Spironolactone is potassium-sparing and causes hyperkalemia. Avoid K+ supplements, K+-rich foods, and salt substitutes (contain KCl).

Chapter 3: Respiratory Medications

1. Answer: B — Recognize that asthma is not well controlled

Rationale: Needing SABA more than 2 times per week (excluding exercise pre-treatment) indicates poorly controlled asthma requiring therapy reassessment.

2. Answer: B — To prevent oral candidiasis

Rationale: Inhaled corticosteroids deposit in the mouth and can cause fungal overgrowth (thrush). Rinsing and spitting prevents this.

3. Answer: C — Salmeterol (Serevent)

Rationale: LABAs have a BLACK BOX WARNING—must NEVER be used alone for asthma due to increased risk of asthma-related death. Always combine with ICS.

4. Answer: B — Use albuterol first, wait 5 minutes, then use fluticasone

Rationale: SABA opens airways first, allowing better penetration of the inhaled corticosteroid.

5. Answer: B — Dry mouth

Rationale: Anticholinergics block muscarinic receptors, reducing secretions and causing dry mouth as the most common adverse effect.

6. Answer: B — Caffeine

Rationale: Theophylline is a methylxanthine, same class as caffeine. Combined use increases adverse effects (tachycardia, insomnia, nervousness).

7. Answer: B — Rebound congestion

Rationale: Using topical decongestants longer than 3-5 days causes rebound congestion (rhinitis medicamentosa), worsening symptoms.

8. Answer: C — Pseudoephedrine (Sudafed)

Rationale: Pseudoephedrine is an alpha-adrenergic agonist causing vasoconstriction and increased BP. Contraindicated in uncontrolled hypertension.

9. Answer: D — Inhale quickly and deeply

Rationale: DPIs require rapid, forceful inhalation to disperse the powder properly. Unlike MDIs, slow inhalation is ineffective.

10. Answer: C — Use the HandiHaler device to inhale the powder

Rationale: Tiotropium capsules are for inhalation only using the HandiHaler. They should never be swallowed.

11. Answer: C — Acetaminophen overdose

Rationale: Acetylcysteine is the antidote for acetaminophen toxicity, replenishing glutathione to prevent liver damage.

12. Answer: B — I should take this medication every evening

Rationale: Montelukast is a daily maintenance medication taken in the evening. It is not for acute symptoms.

13. Answer: B — They cause anticholinergic effects

Rationale: First-generation antihistamines cross the BBB causing sedation and anticholinergic effects (confusion, urinary retention, constipation)—dangerous in elderly.

14. Answer: C — Shaking the inhaler and pressing while inhaling slowly

Rationale: Proper MDI technique includes shaking, coordinating actuation with slow, deep inhalation, and breath-holding.

15. Answer: C — Add a LABA to the regimen

Rationale: Per stepwise approach, if low-dose ICS is insufficient, add LABA (Step 3) rather than increasing to high-dose ICS or adding oral steroids.

16. Answer: A — You can stop abruptly after a short course like this

Rationale: Short courses of oral corticosteroids (< 2 weeks) can be stopped without tapering. Longer courses require gradual taper.

17. Answer: B — Patient taking phenelzine (an MAOI)

Rationale: Dextromethorphan with MAOIs can cause serotonin syndrome—a potentially fatal drug interaction.

18. Answer: B — Should be used daily even when feeling well

Rationale: ICS are maintenance medications that reduce inflammation over time. They must be used daily for effectiveness, not just when symptomatic.

19. Answer: C — Smoking cessation counseling and support

Rationale: Smoking cessation is the MOST important intervention for COPD—the only intervention proven to slow disease progression.

20. Answer: B — Recognize this as oral candidiasis requiring treatment

Rationale: White patches indicate oral thrush from ICS use. This requires antifungal treatment and reinforcement of mouth rinsing.

Chapter 4: Nervous System Medications

1. Answer: B — It typically takes 2-4 weeks to notice improvement

Rationale: SSRIs require 2-4 weeks for therapeutic effect. Patients must understand this to maintain adherence during initial treatment.

2. Answer: C — Aged cheese

Rationale: MAOIs prevent tyramine breakdown. Aged cheeses contain high tyramine levels, which can cause hypertensive crisis when combined with MAOIs.

3. Answer: B — Serotonin syndrome

Rationale: The triad of mental status changes, autonomic instability, and neuromuscular abnormalities (hyperreflexia, tremor) indicates serotonin syndrome from excessive serotonergic activity.

4. Answer: B — Respiratory rate of 10 breaths/min

Rationale: Benzodiazepines cause CNS and respiratory depression. RR < 12 warrants holding the dose and further assessment.

5. Answer: C — Stop haloperidol and notify provider immediately

Rationale: Severe rigidity, hyperthermia, and altered consciousness indicate neuroleptic malignant syndrome (NMS)—a life-threatening emergency requiring immediate drug discontinuation.

6. Answer: B — Recognize this as lithium toxicity

Rationale: Lithium level of 1.8 mEq/L exceeds therapeutic range (0.6-1.2). Confusion and ataxia indicate moderate toxicity requiring intervention.

7. Answer: B — Maintain consistent salt and fluid intake

Rationale: Lithium levels are affected by sodium and hydration status. Dehydration or low sodium intake increases lithium levels and toxicity risk.

8. Answer: B — White blood cell count regularly

Rationale: Clozapine can cause life-threatening agranulocytosis. Regular WBC/ANC monitoring is mandatory through the REMS program.

9. Answer: B — Chronic kidney disease

Rationale: Meperidine's metabolite (normeperidine) accumulates in renal impairment and causes seizures. Meperidine is contraindicated in kidney disease.

10. Answer: A — Administer naloxone

Rationale: RR of 8 with decreased LOC indicates opioid overdose requiring immediate reversal with naloxone. This is a priority intervention.

11. Answer: B — Practice good oral hygiene to prevent gum overgrowth

Rationale: Gingival hyperplasia is a common adverse effect of phenytoin. Good oral hygiene and regular dental care help prevent this.

12. Answer: C — I may experience sexual side effects

Rationale: Sexual dysfunction (decreased libido, anorgasmia) is a common SSRI side effect and frequent cause of nonadherence.

13. Answer: B — Administer prescribed laxatives and increase fluids

Rationale: Constipation is an expected opioid effect that does NOT resolve with tolerance. It must be actively managed with bowel regimen.

14. Answer: C — Sore throat and fever

Rationale: Sore throat and fever may indicate agranulocytosis or aplastic anemia—serious carbamazepine adverse effects requiring immediate evaluation.

15. Answer: B — Flumazenil

Rationale: Flumazenil is the specific benzodiazepine antagonist. Naloxone reverses opioids; acetylcysteine treats acetaminophen overdose.

16. Answer: B — The combination increases CNS depression and can be fatal

Rationale: Alcohol and benzodiazepines both cause CNS depression. Combined use significantly increases risk of respiratory depression and death.

17. Answer: B — Weight gain and hyperglycemia

Rationale: Second-generation antipsychotics, especially olanzapine, cause metabolic syndrome: weight gain, hyperglycemia, and hyperlipidemia.

18. Answer: B — There is increased risk of mortality in this population

Rationale: All antipsychotics carry BLACK BOX WARNING for increased mortality in elderly patients with dementia-related psychosis.

19. Answer: A — High-protein meals taken with the medication

Rationale: High-protein meals compete with levodopa for absorption. Protein should be distributed throughout the day, not taken with medication.

20. Answer: B — Right upper quadrant pain and jaundice

Rationale: Acetaminophen hepatotoxicity presents with RUQ pain, jaundice, elevated liver enzymes, and can progress to liver failure.

Chapter 5: Endocrine Medications

1. Answer: B — 12:00 PM (noon)

Rationale: NPH insulin peaks at 4-12 hours after administration. Given at 7:00 AM, peak effect occurs around noon, when hypoglycemia risk is highest.

2. Answer: B — Hold metformin before and for 48 hours after the procedure

Rationale: IV contrast can cause kidney injury. Metformin is held to prevent lactic acidosis if renal function declines after contrast.

3. Answer: B — I will take this medication on an empty stomach in the morning

Rationale: Levothyroxine absorption is decreased by food, calcium, and iron. Take on empty stomach 30-60 minutes before eating.

4. Answer: B — Decrease the dose gradually as prescribed

Rationale: Long-term corticosteroids suppress the HPA axis. Abrupt discontinuation can cause life-threatening adrenal crisis. Must taper gradually.

5. Answer: B — Give 4 oz of orange juice

Rationale: For conscious patients with hypoglycemia, give 15g fast-acting carbohydrate (juice, glucose tablets) immediately per Rule of 15.

6. Answer: C — Genital yeast infections

Rationale: SGLT2 inhibitors cause glucose to spill into urine (glucosuria), creating an environment that promotes yeast infections.

7. Answer: B — Recognize and treat hypoglycemia symptoms

Rationale: Sulfonylureas stimulate insulin release and can cause hypoglycemia. Patients must recognize symptoms and know how to treat.

8. Answer: B — Remain upright for at least 30 minutes after taking

Rationale: Bisphosphonates can cause severe esophageal irritation. Remaining upright prevents reflux and esophageal damage.

9. Answer: B — Sore throat and fever

Rationale: Sore throat and fever may indicate agranulocytosis, a rare but serious adverse effect of methimazole requiring immediate evaluation.

10. Answer: B — Draw regular first, then NPH

Rationale: "Clear before cloudy"—draw regular (clear) first to prevent NPH (cloudy) from contaminating the regular insulin vial.

11. Answer: B — Metformin increases insulin sensitivity and is first-line therapy

Rationale: Metformin is first-line for Type 2 diabetes because it improves insulin sensitivity, has cardiovascular benefits, and low hypoglycemia risk.

12. Answer: B — Increasing the steroid dose temporarily

Rationale: Stress (illness, surgery, trauma) increases cortisol needs. Patients on chronic steroids need increased doses during stress to prevent adrenal crisis.

13. Answer: C — Regular (Humulin R)

Rationale: Only regular insulin can be given IV. Other insulins are formulated for SubQ use only and cannot be administered intravenously.

14. Answer: B — Explain this often improves with continued use

Rationale: GI side effects (nausea) with GLP-1 agonists typically improve over time. Starting at low doses and titrating slowly helps.

15. Answer: B — It has no peak and provides 24-hour coverage

Rationale: Insulin glargine is "peakless" with steady 24-hour duration, providing basal coverage. Can be given any consistent time daily.

16. Answer: C — New onset shortness of breath and leg edema

Rationale: TZDs cause fluid retention and can precipitate or worsen heart failure. New dyspnea and edema require immediate evaluation.

17. Answer: B — Wear a medical alert bracelet

Rationale: Patients with Addison's disease need lifelong hormone replacement and require stress dosing. Medical alert identification is essential for emergencies.

18. Answer: C — Personal history of medullary thyroid cancer

Rationale: GLP-1 agonists carry BLACK BOX WARNING for thyroid C-cell tumors. Contraindicated in patients with personal/family history of medullary thyroid cancer or MEN2.

19. Answer: B — Nausea and vomiting

Rationale: GI effects, especially nausea, are the most common side effects of GLP-1 agonists including semaglutide. Usually improve with time.

20. Answer: B — Administer glucagon or IV dextrose

Rationale: Unconscious patients cannot swallow safely. Give glucagon IM/SubQ or IV dextrose. Never give oral glucose to unconscious patients.

Chapter 6: Gastrointestinal Medications

1. Answer: B — 30-60 minutes before breakfast

Rationale: PPIs need to be activated by acid. Taking before meals when acid production begins ensures maximum effectiveness.

2. Answer: B — Hypomagnesemia

Rationale: Long-term PPI use can cause hypomagnesemia, leading to muscle cramps, tremors, and cardiac arrhythmias. Monitor magnesium levels.

3. Answer: C — Ondansetron

Rationale: Ondansetron (5-HT3 antagonist) is first-line for chemotherapy-induced nausea due to high effectiveness and favorable side effect profile.

4. Answer: B — Limit use to 12 weeks due to movement disorder risk

Rationale: Metoclopramide carries BLACK BOX WARNING for tardive dyskinesia. Use should not exceed 12 weeks except in rare cases.

5. Answer: B — Take it with a full glass of water

Rationale: Bulk-forming laxatives absorb water. Without adequate fluid, they can cause intestinal obstruction.

6. Answer: C — Senna (Senokot)

Rationale: Stimulant laxatives like senna are recommended for opioid-induced constipation. Docusate alone is often ineffective. Psyllium may worsen OIC.

7. Answer: B — Loperamide (Imodium)

Rationale: Antidiarrheals should not be used with infectious diarrhea (fever, bloody stools)—they can trap bacteria and worsen infection.

8. Answer: B — One hour before meals on an empty stomach

Rationale: Sucralfate requires an acidic environment to form its protective coating. Food and other medications interfere with activation.

9. Answer: B — Black stools are an expected effect

Rationale: Bismuth causes harmless black discoloration of tongue and stools. This is not blood and should not cause alarm.

10. Answer: C — Infliximab

Rationale: TNF-alpha inhibitors like infliximab require TB screening before initiation due to reactivation risk. BLACK BOX WARNING for serious infections.

11. Answer: B — Is pregnant

Rationale: Misoprostol is CONTRAINDICATED in pregnancy—causes uterine contractions and can induce abortion. BLACK BOX WARNING.

12. Answer: B — Apply it behind the ear and wash hands after

Rationale: Scopolamine is applied behind the ear for optimal absorption. Wash hands to avoid getting medication in eyes (causes pupil dilation).

13. Answer: A — Two to three soft stools daily

Rationale: Lactulose draws ammonia into the colon for excretion. The goal is 2-3 soft stools daily to eliminate ammonia effectively.

14. Answer: B — I must complete the full course of all medications

Rationale: H. pylori eradication requires completing the entire regimen (usually 14 days) to prevent resistance and treatment failure.

15. Answer: A — Expect orange-yellow discoloration of urine

Rationale: Sulfasalazine causes harmless orange-yellow discoloration of urine and body fluids. This is expected, not concerning.

16. Answer: B — Dilution and slow administration due to tissue damage risk

Rationale: Promethazine causes severe tissue necrosis with extravasation. Give deep IM or dilute IV and administer slowly.

17. Answer: B — Take on an empty stomach 30 minutes before breakfast

Rationale: Linaclotide is taken on an empty stomach at least 30 minutes before the first meal of the day for optimal effect.

18. Answer: C — Muscle cramps and tremors

Rationale: Muscle cramps and tremors suggest hypomagnesemia, a serious long-term complication of PPI therapy requiring evaluation.

19. Answer: B — With meals and snacks

Rationale: Pancrelipase replaces digestive enzymes and must be taken with food to aid digestion. Without food, there is nothing to digest.

20. Answer: B — Constipation

Rationale: Aluminum-containing antacids cause constipation. Memory aid: Aluminum = constipAtion, Magnesium = Moves things along.

Chapter 7: Anti-Infective Medications

1. Answer: B — Stop the infusion, give antihistamine, and restart at slower rate

Rationale: Red Man Syndrome is rate-related, not a true allergy. Stop infusion, give diphenhydramine, then restart at a slower rate.

2. Answer: B — Nephrotoxicity and ototoxicity

Rationale: Aminoglycosides are notorious for nephrotoxicity (kidney damage) and ototoxicity (hearing loss/vestibular damage). Monitor renal function and hearing.

3. Answer: B — Report any tendon pain immediately

Rationale: Fluoroquinolones carry BLACK BOX WARNING for tendon rupture, especially Achilles tendon. Report tendon pain immediately and stop medication.

4. Answer: B — Alcohol

Rationale: Metronidazole causes a disulfiram-like reaction with alcohol—severe nausea, vomiting, flushing. Avoid alcohol during and 3 days after therapy.

5. Answer: C — Doxycycline

Rationale: Tetracyclines (including doxycycline) are contraindicated in children < 8 years due to permanent tooth staining and bone growth effects.

6. Answer: A — Stopping early can lead to antibiotic resistance

Rationale: Incomplete courses allow surviving bacteria to develop resistance. Full course completion is essential for effective treatment and preventing resistance.

7. Answer: C — Corticosteroids

Rationale: Fluoroquinolone + corticosteroid significantly increases tendon rupture risk. This combination should be avoided when possible.

8. Answer: B — Orange-red discoloration of body fluids

Rationale: Rifampin causes harmless orange-red discoloration of urine, sweat, tears, and other body fluids. This is expected, not concerning.

9. Answer: B — Elevated serum creatinine

Rationale: Amphotericin B is highly nephrotoxic. Elevated creatinine indicates kidney damage requiring dose adjustment or alternative therapy.

10. Answer: A — Check for allergies to penicillin and cephalosporins

Rationale: Always assess allergy history before giving penicillin. Cross-reactivity with cephalosporins exists, especially with severe penicillin allergy.

11. Answer: B — Vitamin B6 (pyridoxine)

Rationale: Isoniazid depletes pyridoxine and causes peripheral neuropathy. Vitamin B6 supplementation prevents this adverse effect.

12. Answer: B — Increase fluid intake to prevent crystalluria

Rationale: Sulfonamides can crystallize in urine. Adequate hydration (2-3 L/day) prevents crystalluria and kidney damage.

13. Answer: B — I will complete all 5 days of the Z-pack

Rationale: Antibiotic courses must be completed as prescribed to prevent resistance, even if the patient feels better before finishing.

14. Answer: D — 25 mcg/mL

Rationale: Vancomycin trough levels > 20 mcg/mL significantly increase nephrotoxicity risk. Level of 25 requires holding and provider notification.

15. Answer: C — Voriconazole

Rationale: Voriconazole can cause visual disturbances including altered color perception and photophobia. Monitor visual function during therapy.

16. Answer: C — Ceftriaxone

Rationale: Patients with severe (anaphylactic) penicillin allergy should avoid cephalosporins due to cross-reactivity risk, especially first-generation cephalosporins.

17. Answer: B — Assessing baseline hearing and renal function

Rationale: Aminoglycosides cause nephrotoxicity and ototoxicity. Baseline assessment allows comparison to detect early toxicity.

18. Answer: B — Hepatotoxicity

Rationale: Azole antifungals including fluconazole are hepatotoxic. Monitor liver function tests during therapy.

19. Answer: B — Oral vancomycin or fidaxomicin is the treatment

Rationale: C. difficile is treated with ORAL vancomycin or fidaxomicin (stays in GI tract). IV vancomycin does not reach the colon effectively.

20. Answer: B — Drink plenty of fluids to protect kidneys

Rationale: Acyclovir can precipitate in renal tubules causing nephrotoxicity. Adequate hydration helps prevent crystal formation and kidney damage.

Chapter 8: Fluids, Electrolytes, and Renal Medications

1. Answer: B — Potassium

Rationale: Loop diuretics like furosemide cause significant potassium loss. Hypokalemia is the major concern, especially in patients on digoxin.

2. Answer: C — IV push administration ordered

Rationale: IV potassium must NEVER be given by IV push—can cause fatal cardiac arrhythmias. This order requires immediate clarification.

3. Answer: C — 0.9% Normal Saline or Lactated Ringer's

Rationale: Isotonic crystalloids (NS, LR) are used for volume resuscitation in hypovolemic shock. They expand intravascular volume effectively.

4. Answer: B — Potassium-rich foods and salt substitutes

Rationale: Spironolactone is potassium-sparing and causes hyperkalemia. Avoid potassium supplements, K+-rich foods, and salt substitutes (contain KCl).

5. Answer: C — Heart failure with pulmonary edema

Rationale: Mannitol initially pulls fluid INTO the intravascular space. This can worsen pulmonary edema in heart failure. Contraindicated.

6. Answer: B — Restrict fluids and monitor neurologic status

Rationale: Moderate hyponatremia is treated with fluid restriction. Rapid correction with 3% saline can cause osmotic demyelination syndrome.

7. Answer: A — Chvostek's sign (facial twitching with tap)

Rationale: Chvostek's sign (facial muscle twitching when facial nerve is tapped) and Trousseau's sign are classic indicators of hypocalcemia.

8. Answer: B — Stop the infusion and notify the provider

Rationale: Absent DTRs indicate magnesium toxicity. Stop infusion immediately and have calcium gluconate (antidote) ready.

9. Answer: B — Ototoxicity

Rationale: Rapid IV administration of loop diuretics (especially furosemide) can cause ototoxicity. Give over 1-2 minutes.

10. Answer: B — I should use sunscreen when outdoors

Rationale: Thiazide diuretics cause photosensitivity. Patients should use sunscreen and protective clothing when outdoors.

11. Answer: B — With meals

Rationale: Phosphate binders must be taken WITH meals to bind dietary phosphate in the GI tract before it is absorbed.

12. Answer: C — Calcium gluconate

Rationale: Calcium gluconate is given FIRST in severe hyperkalemia with ECG changes—it stabilizes the cardiac membrane while other treatments lower K+.

13. Answer: B — Hypertension

Rationale: ESAs like epoetin alfa can cause hypertension. Monitor BP regularly during therapy.

14. Answer: C — 0.45% Normal Saline

Rationale: Hypernatremia requires free water replacement. Hypotonic solutions like 0.45% NS provide free water to correct elevated sodium.

15. Answer: B — Rise slowly to prevent dizziness

Rationale: Alpha-blockers like tamsulosin cause orthostatic hypotension, especially with the first dose. Rise slowly to prevent falls.

16. Answer: C — Calcium gluconate

Rationale: Calcium gluconate is the antidote for magnesium toxicity. It antagonizes the effects of excess magnesium on the heart.

17. Answer: B — Hypotonic

Rationale: 0.45% NS has lower osmolarity than blood, making it hypotonic. It provides free water and moves into cells.

18. Answer: B — Monitor for bradycardia and hypotension

Rationale: Rapid IV calcium administration can cause bradycardia and hypotension. Give slowly and monitor vital signs.

19. Answer: C — PSA levels may decrease by about 50%

Rationale: Finasteride decreases PSA by approximately 50%. When interpreting PSA results, double the reported value for accuracy.

20. Answer: C — Resolution of peripheral edema

Rationale: Effective diuretic therapy in heart failure results in decreased edema, weight loss, and improved breathing—not weight gain or decreased output.

Chapter 9: Immunologic and Hematologic Medications

1. Answer: B — TB screening is complete

Rationale: TNF inhibitors increase risk of TB reactivation. TB skin test or IGRA must be done before starting therapy. BLACK BOX WARNING.

2. Answer: B — Drug toxicity

Rationale: Tremor (neurotoxicity) and elevated creatinine (nephrotoxicity) are signs of tacrolimus toxicity. Drug level should be checked.

3. Answer: A — Recognize this as an expected side effect

Rationale: Bone pain is a common side effect of G-CSF therapy due to increased bone marrow activity. Can be managed with analgesics.

4. Answer: B — Take on an empty stomach with orange juice

Rationale: Iron is best absorbed on empty stomach. Vitamin C (orange juice) enhances absorption. Avoid antacids and dairy.

5. Answer: C — Stop the transfusion immediately

Rationale: Fever, chills, and flank pain suggest acute hemolytic reaction—a medical emergency. Stop transfusion immediately and maintain IV access.

6. Answer: B — Grapefruit juice

Rationale: Grapefruit juice inhibits CYP3A4, significantly increasing cyclosporine levels and toxicity risk.

7. Answer: B — Prednisone 40 mg daily for 3 weeks

Rationale: High-dose corticosteroid therapy causes immunosuppression. Live vaccines are contraindicated in immunocompromised patients.

8. Answer: C — Intramuscular injection

Rationale: Pernicious anemia involves lack of intrinsic factor, preventing oral B12 absorption. IM injection bypasses the GI tract.

9. Answer: B — WBC count of 2,500/mcL

Rationale: Azathioprine causes bone marrow suppression. Low WBC (normal 4,500-11,000) indicates leukopenia requiring dose adjustment or discontinuation.

10. Answer: B — Recent hemorrhagic stroke

Rationale: Thrombolytics dissolve clots but can cause life-threatening bleeding. Recent hemorrhagic stroke is an absolute contraindication.

11. Answer: B — Stop the infusion and initiate emergency care

Rationale: Difficulty breathing and hypotension during rituximab infusion indicate severe infusion reaction requiring immediate intervention.

12. Answer: C — I can take this medication with antacids

Rationale: Mycophenolate absorption is decreased by antacids. Should be taken on empty stomach, separate from antacids.

13. Answer: B — Administer a test dose

Rationale: Iron dextran can cause anaphylaxis. A test dose is required before full infusion to assess for allergic reaction.

14. Answer: B — Factor VIII concentrate

Rationale: Hemophilia A is factor VIII deficiency. Factor VIII concentrate replaces the missing clotting factor before procedures.

15. Answer: C — Depression and suicidal ideation

Rationale: Interferon therapy can cause significant psychiatric effects including depression and suicidal thoughts. Requires close monitoring.

16. Answer: C — 0.9% Normal Saline

Rationale: Blood products are only compatible with 0.9% NS. Other solutions (LR, dextrose) can cause hemolysis or clotting.

17. Answer: B — Bone marrow suppression

Rationale: Hydroxyurea causes bone marrow suppression. Regular CBC monitoring is essential to detect neutropenia, anemia, or thrombocytopenia.

18. Answer: C — Aminocaproic acid

Rationale: Aminocaproic acid inhibits fibrinolysis and is the antidote for excessive bleeding from thrombolytic therapy.

19. Answer: B — Slow the infusion rate and monitor

Rationale: Headache during IVIG infusion may indicate reaction. Slowing the rate often resolves symptoms. If severe, stop and evaluate.

20. Answer: B — I will report any signs of infection immediately

Rationale: TNF inhibitors increase serious infection risk (BLACK BOX). Patients must report fever, cough, or other infection signs promptly.

Chapter 10: Special Populations and High-Alert Medications

1. Answer: B — Verify the child's weight in kilograms

Rationale: Pediatric doses are calculated based on weight in kilograms (mg/kg). Accurate weight is essential for safe dosing.

2. Answer: B — Question the order based on Beers Criteria

Rationale: Diphenhydramine is on the Beers Criteria list as a potentially inappropriate medication for elderly due to anticholinergic effects and fall risk.

3. Answer: C — ACE inhibitors

Rationale: ACE inhibitors are contraindicated throughout pregnancy—they cause fetal renal damage and oligohydramnios in all trimesters.

4. Answer: B — Have another nurse independently verify the dose

Rationale: Insulin is a high-alert medication requiring independent double checks to prevent potentially fatal dosing errors.

5. Answer: B — Separate them to prevent medication errors

Rationale: LASA (look-alike/sound-alike) medications should be stored separately to prevent confusion and medication errors.

6. Answer: B — Patient on metformin with eGFR of 25 mL/min

Rationale: Metformin is contraindicated when eGFR < 30 mL/min due to lactic acidosis risk. This patient needs medication adjustment.

7. Answer: B — Use acetaminophen instead

Rationale: NSAIDs including ibuprofen should be avoided in pregnancy, especially third trimester. Acetaminophen is the preferred analgesic.

8. Answer: B — Perform comprehensive medication reconciliation

Rationale: Polypharmacy (≥5 medications) increases risk of drug interactions and adverse effects. Reconciliation identifies unnecessary medications.

9. Answer: C — U (for unit)

Rationale: "U" can be misread as "0" or "4", causing 10-fold dosing errors. TJC requires writing out "unit" completely.

10. Answer: B — Assess the patient for harm

Rationale: Patient safety is always the priority. First assess for harm, then report and document the error.

11. Answer: C — All medications including OTC, vitamins, and supplements

Rationale: Complete medication reconciliation includes everything the patient takes—prescriptions, OTC, vitamins, supplements, and herbals.

12. Answer: C — Aspirin

Rationale: Aspirin is contraindicated in children with viral illness due to risk of Reye syndrome, a potentially fatal condition.

13. Answer: B — Decreased renal function prolongs drug elimination

Rationale: Aging decreases GFR and renal blood flow, leading to slower drug elimination and accumulation risk.

14. Answer: B — Use premixed solutions when available

Rationale: Concentrated potassium chloride is a high-alert medication. Premixed solutions reduce compounding errors and are preferred.

15. Answer: B — Switching to heparin or LMWH

Rationale: Warfarin is teratogenic (Category X). Heparin and LMWH do not cross the placenta and are safe anticoagulation options in pregnancy.

16. Answer: C — They require additional safety measures

Rationale: High-alert medications have heightened risk of significant harm. They require extra precautions like double checks and smart pumps.

17. Answer: C — Doxycycline

Rationale: Tetracyclines including doxycycline are contraindicated in children < 8 years due to permanent tooth staining and bone effects.

18. Answer: B — Asking the patient to explain what they learned

Rationale: Teach-back confirms patient understanding by having them explain the information in their own words.

19. Answer: B — Possible adverse drug reaction

Rationale: New confusion in elderly patients on multiple medications should prompt evaluation for adverse drug reaction before assuming other causes.

20. Answer: B — Independent double checks by two nurses

Rationale: Independent double checks are the most effective strategy for catching high-alert medication errors before they reach the patient.

References

Adams, M. P., Urban, C. Q., & El-Hussein, M. T. (2023). Pharmacology: Connections to nursing practice (5th ed.). Pearson.

American Geriatrics Society Beers Criteria Update Expert Panel. (2023). American Geriatrics Society 2023 updated AGS Beers Criteria. Journal of the American Geriatrics Society, 71(7), 2052-2081.

Burchum, J. R., & Rosenthal, L. D. (2022). Lehne's pharmacology for nursing care (11th ed.). Elsevier.

Institute for Safe Medication Practices. (2024). ISMP list of high-alert medications in acute care settings.

National Academies of Sciences, Engineering, and Medicine. (2007). Preventing medication errors. The National Academies Press.

National Council of State Boards of Nursing. (2019). NCSBN Clinical Judgment Measurement Model.

U.S. Food and Drug Administration. (2014). Pregnancy and lactation labeling (drugs) final rule.

Vallerand, A. H., & Sanoski, C. A. (2024). Davis's drug guide for nurses (19th ed.). F.A. Davis Company.

Made in United States
Orlando, FL
04 November 2026

90201047R00092